Hypermobility Without Tears

Moving Pain-Free with Hypermobility and Ehlers-Danlos Syndrome

Copyright © 2019 Jeannie Di Bon
London, United Kingdom
W: www.jeanniedibon.com
E: jeannie@jeanniedibon.com

All Rights Reserved

No part of this book may be reproduced in any form, by photocopying or by electronic or mechanical means, including information storage or retrieval systems, without permission in writing from both the copyright owner and the publisher of this book. This book is not intended to give any medical, legal, media and/or financial advice to the readers.

Other books in this series

Pilates Without Tears – The 5-Step No Pain, No Strain Strategy to Move and Feel Great (2016)

Contents

Acknowledgements……………………………..…….………………….7

About the Author………………………………………….……..……….9

Foreword……………………………………………….…………………11

Why This Book
My Story……………………….....………………………..……………15

Chapter One: Breath
Explore the Integral Breath……………..………………….…………21

Chapter Two: Relaxation
The Key to Health of Body and Mind……………………….……...…31

Chapter Three: Proprioception
From My Head to My Toes, Inside and Out………………..……………39

Chapter Four: Stability
The Elusive Search……………………………………………………57

Chapter Five: Balance
The Daily Challenge……………………………………………………85

Chapter Six: Posture
An Awakening of the Senses..105

Chapter Seven
Practical Improvements with the IMM...127

Further Information..137

References..141

Acknowledgements

I wish to express my heartfelt thanks to a number of people who made this book possible:

- My husband Ilario, for his support, patience and guidance.
- My beautiful sons who keep me smiling and laughing.
- Family and friends for all their encouragement.
- Dr Leslie Russek for taking the time to proof read my book and for writing such a wonderful foreword for the book.
- The Ehlers-Danlos community for inspiring me to express my thoughts and feelings on movement.
- My clients who allow me to love what I do.

I am very grateful to you all.

Thank you.

About the Author

Jeannie Di Bon is a Movement Therapist specializing in working with people with hypermobility, Ehlers-Danlos Syndrome and chronic pain. Originally trained in Pilates, over the past decade her research and study have gone on to encompass biomechanics, anatomy, neuroscience and pain management.

Jeannie has hypermobile Ehlers-Danlos Syndrome and rehabbed her body and mind from chronic pain by developing her own method – the Integral Movement Method. She now shares this approach with her clients worldwide.
Further information on Jeannie's work can be found at www.jeanniedibon.com

She writes regularly on her own blog and for The Mighty, The Huffington Post and Thrive Global on the subject of chronic illness. She presents for The EDS Society and other charities. Jeannie is also an educator of teachers and therapists in the field of hypermobility. Her digital courses – among them, *Movement Strategies for the Hypermobile Client* – have proven very popular.

Jeannie's first book – *Pilates Without Tears*, published in 2016 – continues to be sold internationally, receiving outstanding feedback.

Foreword – by Dr Leslie Russek

Jeannie Di Bon has accomplished something quite impressive: translating personal experience with hypermobility, Pilates training, and years of thoughtful movement practice and teaching into a series of lessons that can help people with hypermobility learn to move and live with less pain. I have been recommending her on-line Pilates course "Strengthen Your Hypermobile Core" to patients for years. I have received excellent feedback from patients, who say that it made them aware of dysfunctional movement patterns that they finally realize that subtle differences in how they breathe, stand and move has profound effects on pain. This book provides the next tool for people with hypermobility to gain better awareness of their bodies, and control of their lives.

Jeannie starts the book with breathing, and for good reason. We do it all the time and usually don't think about how we do it. But dysfunctional breathing can cause tension throughout the core, tension that causes pain and that prevents us from moving correctly. One of Jeannie's great insights is that people with hypermobility often need to learn to relax muscles, not just activate more muscles. It may seem unintuitive that people who are too flexible should learn how to relax. But muscle guarding (or bracing) occurs as a protective mechanism to provide support to lax joints, and this guarding can lead to excessive muscle tone that is not only painful but leads to inappropriate movement patterns. Jeannie challenges the traditional Pilates practice of drawing the abdominal muscles up and in for all core stabilization; constant activation of these muscles makes it difficult to breath and move, and creates excessive tension. People with hypermobility do need to activate muscles for stability, but not all the muscles all the time.

This book also integrates current thinking about pain neuroscience: pain is the brain's response to a sense of danger rather than a measure of tissue damage. People with hypermobility are fearful of movement, either because their bodies are unstable, untrustworthy, or in pain. If the brain can learn to trust the body and trust movement, the perception of danger is decreased and pain can be decreased. Many of the exercises in this book are designed to overcome this fear of movement. New pain science also tells us that neural patterns that perpetuate pain can be changed by modifying thought patterns and movement. Jeannie's approach does both: changes how we move and how we think about movement.

This book will become a valuable resource for people with hypermobility. It allows them to explore new possibilities for living within their hypermobile bodies. It encourages people to listen to their bodies in a non-judgmental way and to develop a new relationship with bodies that have often been untrustworthy, difficult to understand, and the source of great pain. Jeannie's personal journey is an inspiring example of how people with hypermobility can change their lives for the better.

We are fortunate that she has managed to share the insights from her years of struggle, reflection and practice in such a clear and accessible guide.

Dr Leslie Russek PT, DPT, PhD
Orthopaedic Certified Specialist
Professor of Physical Therapy
Clarkson University, New York

Why This Book
My Story

"When you hear hoof beats behind you, don't expect to see a zebra"
T E Woodward, Medical Researcher, 1948

I can still remember the barrage of tests and investigations. The confusion on the doctors' faces, as results were showing no serious underlying condition. That's what they were looking for – I realise that now. They were not looking for a zebra. They were trained to look for horses – the predictable, easily recognizable. They had probably not even heard of Ehlers-Danlos Syndrome (EDS) back in 1983. Medical students today still receive little training or information about connective tissue disorders like EDS. In 1983, I was 13 years old and after the stress of my parents' divorce, I had started suffering severe digestive issues. After a few months, the doctors announced I had Irritable Bowel Syndrome (IBS). I've lost count of the number of times a doctor has told me it's all down to IBS and instructed me to eat more fibre and try Pilates or yoga to relax. Dismissive in its nature and kind of ironic now, as I trained to become a Pilates teacher in 2008.

Hypermobility Without Tears

Looking back over 30 years later, I see this original stress was the trigger for this connective tissue disorder, EDS. Like many people with this condition, the IBS diagnosis was just the start of a long list of 'unrelated' medical conditions over the years. Crippling knee pain put a stop to my county level cross-country running, chronic back and shoulder pain became a constant feature. I felt old and tired in my twenties. Unexplained stretch marks and wounds that wouldn't heal, leaving strange looking scars behind. I remember being scorned by a local doctor when I asked why I was suffering from random bruising, that I had no recollection of causing myself. Somewhere deep in my mind, this lack of answers was causing me stress and worry, but I tried to forget and carry on with my life.

Things did settle for a while – I think I just put up with daily migraines and a jaw that would lock shut overnight. I married and looked forward to starting a family. I discovered then the hormonal changes in pregnancy set off a whole new part of my EDS journey: pelvic girdle pain, quick dilations in labour and a postnatal exhaustion I thought all new parents had. But my exhaustion went on for years, I never seemed to have the energy that other mums my age had. They all wanted to go to the park after school and have play dates. I just wanted to crawl home. I craved sleep so badly. Exhaustion finally led to pneumonia – two episodes in quick succession with lengthy hospitalizations.

But you carry on past the sickness, past the diagnosed mitral valve prolapse, the chronic fatigue, past the third pneumonia. The whole host

Why This Book

of medical complaints became quite a list. The years pass by, you think this is just how you are. Deep down I thought there must be a severe illness waiting to be discovered. Surely it was not normal to feel like this.

I wanted to feel in control again of my body and my mind. I was worrying too much about my health. I focused too much on what was wrong with me. In 2007 I found an exercise method that seemed to agree with me. A physiotherapist I was seeing for chronic shoulder and back pain recommended to try Pilates. His exact words were "you are literally hanging off your joints. You have no stability or core strength". I had no idea what he was talking about, but I tried a class. It was gentle, non-impact and also relaxing. There was so much about it I liked – I was soon taking 3 classes a week and in a short space of time, I knew I was going to train to be a teacher and learn as much as I could about movement.

Fast forward 10 years, my physical and mental pain had gone. I'd spent the years teaching thousands of clients and attending courses to learn from some of the world's leading experts in movement and anatomy. I have read almost every book out there on movement theories and philosophies. I had refined and organized all that I had learnt and figured out into a method for my body – the Integral Movement Method (IMM) – that had healed my pain and made me strong for the first time in my life. The best thing was being able to share the method with my clients and a growing client base of people with EDS (it's funny how the universe works sometimes – it brings you the people you are meant to meet and work with) and chronic pain. I started to see this method, which I created to heal my own body, really did work on other people too. My first book *Pilates Without Tears* (2016) examines this method in full detail. (We will review the elements of the IMM in Chapter Seven.)

But, EDS has no rules. It's unpredictable in nature. I knew my symptoms were exacerbated by stress. The sudden death of my mother in 2017 after a cancer battle left me distraught. The stress was just too much for my body to bare. It went into overdrive and the rest of the year was spent battling a little-known condition called Mast Cell Activation Disorder (MCAD). Mast cells are important blood cells in the body for protecting the immune system. In a healthy system, the mast cells act beneficially to protect and heal the body, but with a disorder these same cells trigger inappropriately and can have a negative effect on the body (www.mastcellaction.org). My body was fighting everything – my autoimmune system was wrecked. My consultant then diagnosed EDS. I cried tears of relief. Like many of you reading this story, the frustration of not being heard for so many years causes distress and pain. I finally had confirmation of something I had felt all along - I too was a zebra. This empowered me further to continue to spread awareness and knowledge of the power of movement therapy. This is how this book has come to fruition, for which I am so grateful to have this opportunity.

I wanted to share my personal journey with you because I know it is not extraordinary. It is a common journey for those with EDS and

Why This Book

hypermobility disorders. I understand the pain and frustration you may have experienced over the years. I've known the fear and isolation of not knowing what to do, how to improve my health and experiencing a lack of understanding in the medical, health and fitness industry. Over ten years of self-exploration, searching for answers and solutions led me to movement therapy. Movement therapy was the key to my return to health. There is currently little research in this field: there is one paper – "The Pilates client on the hypermobility spectrum" (McNeil et al, 2017) – examining the impact of Pilates on EDS, but this was with a study sample of just one client. There is however research into the impact of Pilates on various issues which highlights benefits that could also positively impact people with hypermobility. A recent study by Byers et al (2017) found that "Pilates has demonstrated efficacy as a tool for the rehabilitation of a wide range of conditions". This is useful information, as we know that EDS and hypermobility come with a vast array of conditions and co-morbidities. In a further recent study by Cruz-Diaz et al in 2017, they found that twelve weeks of Pilates intervention were effective in reducing pain intensity and improving disability, fear of movement and improving deep trunk muscle thickness.

This book is structured to allow you to follow my method as I do. It shares the path I take all my hypermobility clients on and opens the door to pain-free, confident movement, without fear and anxiety. I truly hope it will serve its purpose for those with hypermobility to begin moving, to discover a new approach to exercise. The book is easy to read and follow, with practical exercises along the way. Chapter One invites us to examine our breathing patterns and the implications on our health. Chapter Two turns attention to the mind body connection – how we can unravel tension and stress that may be holding us back. Chapter Three examines the role of proprioception and leads into its partner, Stability, in Chapter Four. Balance is essential for everyday life and Chapter Five will delve deeper into this topic. The No Pain, No Strain evolution is explained in Chapter Six. By Chapter Seven we are ready to demonstrate how the Integral Movement Method can help with hypermobility and EDS.

My message to you through this book is that there is hope. No matter what your previous story, take heart that every small physical step is a huge emotional one. Through small steps, you will grow in confidence. Enjoy this journey. It's personal to you. We are all unique, there is no right or wrong to seek but simply the enjoyment of moving well and feeling connected to our body and mind.

Yours in movement.

Jeannie Di Bon

Chapter One: Breath
Explore the Integral Breath

"Do not be tense when you inhale. Do not get involved, receive the air in a passive, detached way, as though you were only an observer, an outsider."
Vanda Scaravelli, Yogi, 1991

It is our first act of life and our last. Breath is our very essence. We breathe an average of 12-20 breaths a minute, over 23,000 a day. Yet we often take this for granted. Until we become sick – and those with EDS often suffer respiratory illnesses from colds, bronchitis, bronchiectasis, asthma and pneumonia. A study in 2007 (Morgan et al) found that there was a "significant increase in the frequency of a wide range of respiratory symptoms and reduced exercise tolerance" in subjects with EDS and hypermobility compared to control subjects.

From a pure health perspective, it makes sense therefore to learn to maximize our breathing capacity. Much of our lung tissue is situated in the back of the body – but do we ever breathe there?

Hypermobility Without Tears

Aside from the respiratory health benefits that relearning to breathe effectively can give us, the breath holds much information about our state of mind, our movement patterns often driven by fear and guarding. When we have been in pain, maybe chronic pain for many years, we often adopt a subconscious guarding pattern. We internally brace in anticipation of the pain we are expecting. We subconsciously believe these holding patterns are protecting us from future pain and that they are serving us well. It is well known that for some people in chronic, persistent pain they need only to think about a movement and it produces pain. Your brain is very good at protecting you from anything it may perceive as dangerous to your tissue. Scientific research has discovered that thought processes can be powerful enough to maintain a 'pain state' (Butler et al, 2003). This is a misconception on the brain's behalf. It is in over-protection mode, understandably. It knows the past pain experiences you have had and wants to help you avoid more. This is called over sensitization. We become so sensitive to the pain signals that even the slightest of movements is considered a potential damaging threat by the brain. But within these holding patterns live tension, bracing and pain. Yes, pain. By bracing, we are restricting free, fluid movement of the body, which in turn causes further pain. By trying so hard to avoid pain, we actually create a situation that potentially causes more of it.

A client recently explained how it is possible to remove these bracing patterns:

Chapter One: Breath

"The blend of mindful and focused movement is allowing me to listen to my body again. In just two sessions, through visualisations, along with careful control of the body I am very encouraged by how much I am already able to release the tension and bracing that has become a common daily feature for me"
Henry, Client with Hypermobile EDS

With my own body and that of my clients, I have discovered that relearning to breathe is the first step to success. It's something all of us can do, regardless of ability. This is great news.

Faulty breathing patterns can also cause pain in the thoracic area. According to the leading pain expert Dr Pradeep Chopra, there is a lack of proprioception in EDS patients between the ribs, diaphragm, lungs and other breathing muscles. This abnormal pattern can be enough to cause pain and the feeling of not being able to take a full breath. This gives us another reason to spend time getting to know our breath and current habits.

To recap, five reasons why conscious breathing is important for hypermobility:

1) Respiratory health
2) Pain relief

3) Recognition of bracing and holding patterns
4) Improvement of proprioception in the thorax
5) Relaxation benefits

Let's get started with some simple practical exercises for conscious breathing.

EXERCISE - Recognize the Guarding

If you have spent many years unaware of your breath, how do we know what guarding feels like?

I know from experience of working with hundreds of clients with hypermobility and EDS that it is very common practice. But it is a changeable habit – that's all it is. A habit that we have adopted due to our circumstances. Once you are aware of your habits, you can change them. Nothing is set in stone.

This first exercise is best performed lying on your back, knees bent.

Chapter One: Breath

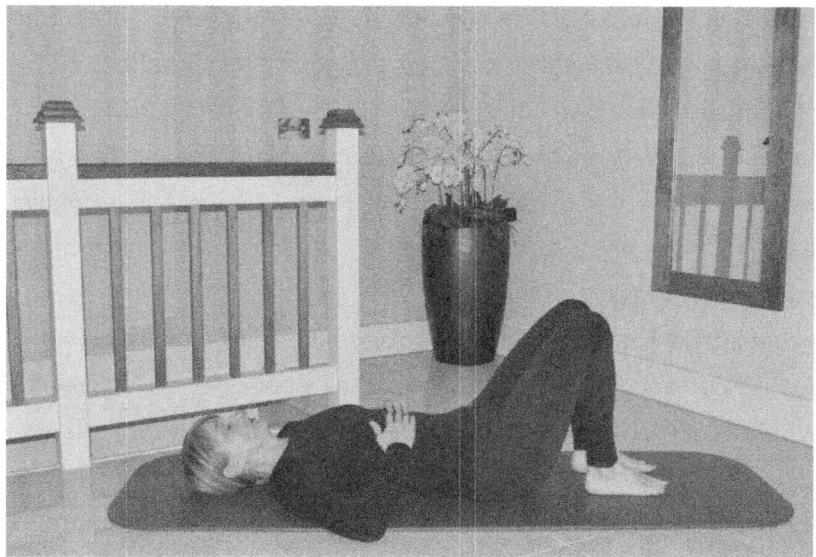

Rest your hands on the front of your rib cage and notice the weight of your hands there.

Spend a few moments simply noticing your breath. Don't try to change or control it. Simply observe the breath enter your body and notice it leave. Notice the flow, the rhythm, the depth.

Observe. When you exhale, what happens? Does the breath leave the body fully? Do you have to force the breath out? Does it feel like it's stuck in your chest or throat?

As you become a passive observer of your breath, notice the mind has quietened. This is where stress and anxiety can begin to unwind. Stress

Hypermobility Without Tears

is reflected in our breath. Try to notice the exhale and what it gives your body. As your breath leaves the body, can you start to feel the weightiness of your own body? Imagine you are lying on a foam mattress and every out-breath causes you to sink further into the mattress. You sink so deep that when you stand there will be an imprint on the mattress of your body, your spine. Can you see the shape of your bones? Would one side of the body be heavier? Would there be a deeper imprint in some areas? Do you see a balance of your imprint – are the head and pelvis weighing the same? What does the alignment look like – did you lie straight on the mattress?

We are seeking a softening of the body, a surrender to the ground. The weight of your body sinks to the back. You feel your organs weighted down underneath you. As the body softens, it lengthens and widens. You are creating space, spinal elongation and joint space with your breath. Your imprint has changed shape again.

Even when we think we are still, we are not. The breath will cause the body to change and morph, to lengthen and spread. Our job is to be patient enough to allow and observe this as it happens.
By allowing your body to sink and soften, you began to work with gravity rather than fighting it. Gravity is your movement friend. When we start to foster the relationship between our breath, our body and the ground, we start to surrender any unnecessary tension in the body and mind. We start to feel secure, supported, grounded – all the things hypermobility makes challenging.

Chapter One: Breath

The back of the ribcage is able to rest heavily on the floor, releasing tension from the front of the body. What we want to notice is a softening and dropping of the ribcage on the exhale. Can you feel a downward motion of the ribs on the exhale? The more you focus on the back of the ribs, the easier this becomes. Do not attempt to push the front of the ribs down, as this causes further tension.

Once we have appreciation of the weight of our breath in our thoracic spine, we can move to full body breathing. For a healthy breathing pattern that is not harboring tension, we want to see the belly involved too. Pilates as a practice often cues the drawing up and in of the pelvic floor and lower abdominal muscles. This never sat well with me – it felt unnatural to force this on the body. What I wanted was a body that responded naturally to the breath. I did not want to interfere with the natural patterns. If you have ever tried to suck and draw in the abdominals, hold them that way and then move, you will know how difficult that can be. It feels tense and again a form of bracing we do not need. Due to lack of proprioception – which we will cover in greater detail in Chapter Three – we will recruit more than we need to. This leads to more tension, and I've seen pelvic girdle pain and back pain as a result of this practice.

Understanding of how the diaphragm moves when we are breathing can help too with our breathing patterns. The diaphragm is a large dome-shaped muscle at the base of the lungs and is the most efficient muscle for breathing. With contraction of the diaphragm, the belly expands on inhale, rather than just the sternum or the chest. Your abdominal muscles help move the diaphragm so these should naturally respond to your breath. They should not, therefore, be held or sucked in during the process of inhalation and exhalation, as is so often cued in Pilates and exercise classes.

EXERCISE – Exploring your Breath Moving

Side-lying Breathwork

Lie comfortably on one side with bent knees. You can use cushions or a rolled-up towel to support your head and neck. If possible, place one hand on the top ribcage. Close your eyes and focus on your breath moving in and out of the body. This time, try to feel the air moving up into one side of the body – the ribcage that is exposed to the ceiling. Notice how easy or challenging it is to breathe on the side, allowing the lung to expand. Are there are any tight areas? After 5 minutes, change sides and compare the difference. It is often noticeable that one side is easier to breathe into. This is a really fantastic exercise to encourage the ribcage to move laterally when we breathe. Of course, go gently and do not force the breath – especially if you are prone to ribs that sublux. Slow and gentle is key.

Chapter One: Breath

Prone Breathwork

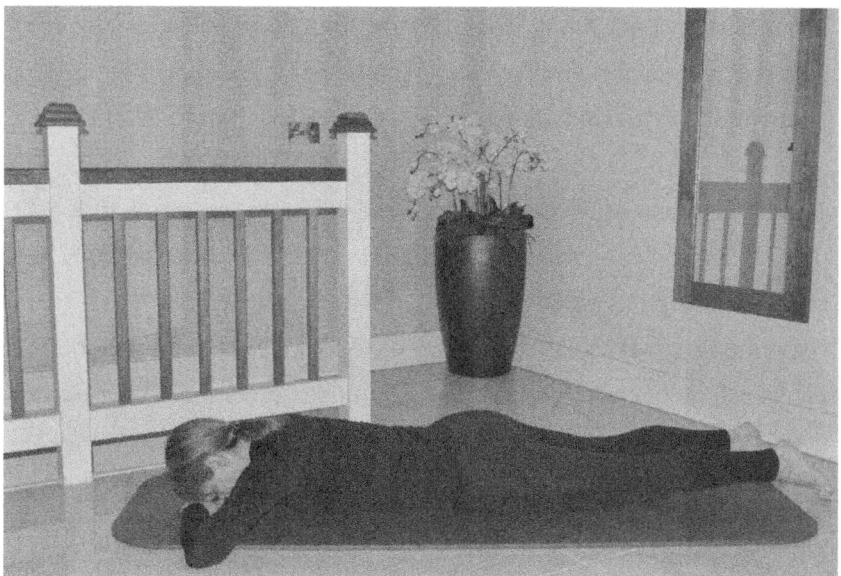

Another way to explore the breath and its impact on the body is to lie prone (face down). Again, use a cushion to support your head or rest your head in your hands. If you experience low back pain when lying on your front, I recommend placing a towel or cushion under the pelvis. This will help alleviate the pain. Now that the front of the ribcage is resting on the floor, it is much easier to send the breath into the back of the body. Imagine you have gills like a fish and as you inhale the gills on your back open. When you exhale, they gently close. This promotes movement and space in the back of the body. This is typically a neglected area for breath – we tend to breathe at the front of the body, especially if we have been in chronic pain.

Hypermobility Without Tears

Exploring this 3-dimensional breathing pattern is really important for creating space in the torso and massaging the connective tissue. The connective tissue can get 'stuck' around the thorax, which can cause pain and restrictions when moving. Gentle breathwork can often be enough to start moving the fascia, thereby allowing freer movements.

This chapter has allowed us to experience the role that gravity has to play on our body and movement patterns. When we allow the body to soften, we begin to work with gravity rather than fighting it. Hypermobility makes us feel that we have to fight just to be upright. In a sense, we do because we have to work much harder than other people due to lack of muscle tonality, control and awareness. These are all areas we are going to work on in future chapters.

Let's continue our journey into Relaxation – a perfect partner for Breath.

Chapter Two: Relaxation
The Key to Health of Body and Mind

"Mindful touch and movement grounds people and allows them to discover tensions that they may have held for so long, they are no longer even aware of them."
Bessel Van Der Kolk, Author – The Body Keeps the Score, 2014

Relaxation follows on beautifully from the subject of Breath. If you completed the breathing exercises in Chapter One, you may have experienced this intertwined relationship already. The simple act of focusing on the breath even for a few minutes is an instant de-stressor and engages the relaxation response in the body. Deeper, connected breathing creates deeper feelings within the body because it creates movement from within (J Stirk 2015).

The relaxation response first cited by Herbert Benson MD at Harvard Medical School found the benefits of regular breathing practice and meditation were physiological changes like slowing of breathing rate and release of muscle tension. This is exactly what our body needs if we have been stressed and anxious due to our EDS symptoms. This approach to movement has been proven to be beneficial with stress-related conditions.

We learnt in the previous chapter that bracing and guarding is a common feature for those with EDS and hypermobility. It makes sense that this pattern creates tension and anxiety in the body and mind. Research has also shown that those with these conditions tend to suffer with anxiety more. A recent article by Dr Hakim (2018) stated "anxiety disorders and other psychological concerns are present to higher degrees in hEDS/HSD than other conditions."

Anxiety and stress are a normal response for someone who may have been in chronic and often unexplained pain for many years. It is also a normal response if you are fearful about movement – maybe because of the pain itself, of injuring yourself or creating a flare-up. Past bad exercise experiences will be stored in your nervous system and the brain will be happy to trigger those thoughts, feelings and experiences at the mere thought of exercising again. Sensitization is at play.

Imagine if those records stored in the brain that create those fears and anxieties could be overwritten. Imagine erasing that data, reprogramming your nervous system so that it had a totally new approach to movement. When you thought of movement, it would not fill you with dread and fear, but pleasurable sensations and the knowledge that you are doing something good for your body and yourself. It is so important that we remember "the amount of pain you experience does

Chapter Two: Relaxation

not necessarily relate to the amount of tissue damage you have sustained" (Butler et al, 2003). If you have ever sustained a paper cut on your finger, can you recall how painful that can be and yet the cut is tiny? On the other side, you hear stories of athletes continuing to play games of rugby and football with broken bones and they do not feel a thing. This is because the brain is distracted – it is not listening to the pain signals and is motivated by the pleasure the individual has in playing sport. If there is no pain, it means that the tissue changes are not perceived by the brain as a threat. What we need to do is to train our brain to feel that movement is not a threat, so that this too can become pain free and enjoyable. To do this, we have to start with the mind-body relationship.

I call this the 'Unwind' stage in my Integral Movement Method (IMM). It is absolutely possible to unwind tension and fear held within the body, which can reflect itself in movement restrictions, pain and stiffness. It is an essential element to unwind thoughts that no longer serve us well and replace them. How do we do that? By showing the mind that nothing bad is going to happen when we move. By reminding the mind that our bodies love movement and that we are designed to move. Our body has 360 joints – that's 360 moving parts. If we have that many moving surfaces, surely they are meant to move as opposed to be inactive day after day. Of course, one of the issues our hypermobile bodies have is that those moving surfaces can move too much, causing pain, subluxations and dislocations. But if we trained our body awareness, proprioception and control so that the supporting muscles and ligaments helped those joints, that could really help. That's what we will be looking at in the future chapters.

To start the Unwind process I have found that the most successful route is to work on the mind first and then the body. I would see little point in starting to work on strength and connection physically with movement and exercise if the mind were not willing or able at that stage to participate and let down those over protective barriers. I need to desensitize the body I am working with before we attempt movement.

My client explains how this approach can work:

"Being hypermobile, I have suffered pain and injury all my life. It is only through Jeannie's work that I have come to know a life that is physically pain-free."
Sarah, Client, Hypermobile EDS

The breathing exercises are a fantastic way to start this Unwind process and begin the much-needed relaxation response. Observing the breath is a simple form of meditation. Meditation is often thought of as some weird practice that means you need to clear your mind of all thoughts. That is not the case. The act of observing the breath is meditation. Research has proven the impact meditation can have on pain signals from the brain to the body (Harvard Medical School – A Mind-body approach to pain management and wellness, 2018). Meditation can be deemed as a wakeful or conscious hypometabolic (low metabolic rate)

Chapter Two: Relaxation

integrated state in which you are more deeply at rest than during sleep. If you suffer with poor sleep hygiene, this is a comforting thought. It stops me worrying about a poor night's sleep quite so much as I can restore during my meditation practice.

I teach my clients meditation and practice it daily myself. I find it calming and helps focus the mind. It helps clear the brain fog too that EDS sometimes brings. Remember it is a practice. It does not have to be perfect. If your mind wanders, that's normal. The art is to catch yourself and bring your thoughts back to your breath. Over time, you may find your thoughts wander less and your mind can rest. When you've been in chronic pain, having a mind that is distracted away from the pain and our condition for even ten minutes a day is a huge progress. Our mind needs rest as much as our body to begin healing.

Contemporary neuroscience states that our sense of ourselves is anchored in a vital connection with our bodies. Therefore, we do not truly know ourselves unless we can feel and interpret our physical sensations (B Van Der Kolk, 2014). This is why my method focuses so deeply on the building of sensory awareness – vital for our proprioceptive senses.

EXERCISE – Simple Meditation Practice

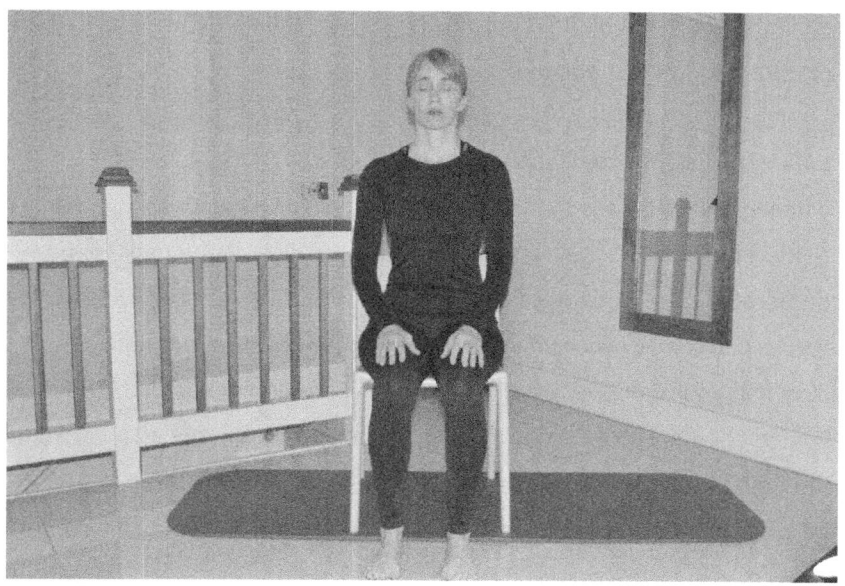

Firstly, you need to choose a special word or phrase. Something that means something to you. It could be a religious phrase, or a declaration of love or a simple word like "rest", "heal" or "love".
Sit on a chair with feet firmly placed on the ground. Palms resting on your thighs face down.

Close your eyes softly and quietly watch your breath inhale and exhale, without trying to control or change it. Feel your body soften into the chair, your feet heavy on the ground. Feel the pull of gravity down into the chair.

Chapter Two: Relaxation

Take a slow inhale. On the exhale say your chosen word or phrase to yourself.
Repeat this process for 10 minutes. You can set a timer, but this can cause distraction and anxiety as you wait for the timer to go off. If you can learn to gage how long 10 minutes is for yourself, you will have more control.

When your time is complete, slowly open the eyes. Sit for a further minute observing your breath.

You can of course spend longer than 10 minutes. A beginner would practice up to 20 minutes.

Now that we have spent some time calming the mind, allowing it to be more responsive and welcoming to new movement practice, we can move on to explore the role of Proprioception.

Chapter Three: Proprioception
From My Head to My Toes, Inside and Out

"Fascia constitutes a body-wide tensional network, which serves as our richest and most important sensory organ for feeling changes in our own body."
Robert Schliep, PhD, Director of Fascia Research Project, 2015

According to the Collins English Dictionary, proprioception is defined as "the neurological ability of the body to sense movement and position". ScienceDirect describe it as "the unconscious or conscious awareness of joint position".

Words that reach out to me are '*sense*' and '*awareness*'. I work with my clients on building sensory awareness for this very reason – it helps tremendously with our proprioceptive abilities.

But why do hypermobile bodies have such a hard time with proprioception? Proprioception is the kinesthetic sense that enables us to sense the relative position of the parts of our body, our posture, our balance and movement. We know that this sense is often lacking in those with hypermobility. There has been research into this by Clayton et al (2015) but they also state that no one yet knows why it is lacking in hypermobile people. This lack of awareness means that we are not aware when we have locked our joints, for example. When we lock joints, this action places pressure on the joint and surrounding structures leading to wear and tear and a greater chance of injury. With a locked joint, the muscles no longer have to work to support us. In turn, they become deconditioned and weaker. With deconditioned tissue, pain increases. The often unconscious act of locking joints sets off a spiral of dysfunction and pain. On top of this, proprioceptive deficit can make us more accident-prone, clumsy and prone to running into things. Propensity for bruising, cuts and sprains are then increased.

This lack of proprioceptive awareness also means we can move into ranges well beyond what is considered 'normal'. Maybe you were able to do 'party tricks' to amuse your friends. Maybe you assumed that was normal. I had no idea people's fingers could not bend backwards like mine for years. For me, that was normal. It does not hurt to do it, so why would it be wrong? But it is another habit that does not serve us well. It promotes range of movement that we need to be reigning in. Repeated overstretching to that degree will only exacerbate the laxity and the chances of the joints slipping out of place (Jason Parry, Clinical Specialist Physiotherapist, UCL, 2017).

Chapter Three: Proprioception

Although there is yet to be a definitive answer as to why hypermobility causes a lack of proprioception, I wanted to introduce the role of fascia here and its very special role in this field. Here's an extract from my blog in April 2018 (posted on my website), which will help explain the role of fascia for hypermobility.

"Fascia is a three-dimensional sheet of internal connective tissue in our bodies the covers everything; wrapping around muscles, bones, organs, vessels and the nervous system. It separates different layers of tissue, preventing friction, and has been likened to a cling-film that protects the various elements of your body.

It also has an elastic quality, contracting and expanding, and stores and releases the kinetic energy from our body's movement. Fascia is the biggest sensory organ in the whole body – which is why I believe building sensory awareness in our bodies is crucial to healthy movement. It helps prevent or minimise stress to a local muscle and it protects the integrity of the whole body.

Our fascia plays a fundamental role in proprioception, which is our ability to know where we are in the space around us and sense movement within our joints. Proprioception also allows our body to respond to our environment more quickly than our conscious mind. Those in the hypermobile community may be aware that they lack these full capabilities, but may not be entirely sure why. The reason is that fascia has 10 times more proprioceptors than muscle (Myers 2011).

Hypermobility Without Tears

This can pose a problem for EDS sufferers as fascia is made up of dense bundles of collagen – and genetic collagen defects have been found for all but one type of EDS. So, if our collagen-based fascia isn't fully functioning as it should, then it appears that our proprioception could be affected too.

[Note: since this article was written, research by the Ehlers-Danlos Society has been underway to understand the genetic code responsible for hypermobile EDS. It is not yet known.]

Because fascia is everywhere, and because EDS and hypermobility sufferers have genetic collagen problems [see note above regarding hEDS]*, it can mean that those with the condition can feel it affects anywhere in the body – from the heart and lungs to digestion, muscles and joints. And because it is everywhere, this is how that myofascial pain we experience seems to spread around the body, often with no particular pattern or reason. It is transmitted through the fascia".*

You can read the full article at https://jeanniedibon.com/blog/

Recent research appears to back up this theory too, which is encouraging for our own understanding. A paper by Robert Schliep in 2015 looked at the role of fascia as a sensory organ and confirmed that "fascia has important roles in proprioception, interoception (subconscious signaling in the body), and nociception (the ability to feel pain). He explains that in the past much emphasis has been placed on the joint receptors in the joint capsules, but research is now indicating

Chapter Three: Proprioception

that fascia could potentially be more important due to the rich density of proprioceptive nerve endings. It would appear the scientific field is moving towards the fact that fascia constitutes our most important perceptual organ (Schliep, 2015).

To recap, why is improving our proprioception going to be an important part of a movement therapy program?

1. It decreases injury - less strain and sprains.
2. It decreases wear and tear on joints.
3. It improves coordination and clumsiness decreases.
4. It improves whole body sensory awareness.
5. It promotes fluid movement with fascia friendly strategy.

Let's start working on our proprioception.

We have actually already started with our breathing exercises. You are now more aware of the physiological and emotional impact your breath has on your body. You've had a felt sense of the weight of your body sinking into the floor. Proprioception between the diaphragm, ribs and breathing muscles has already improved. Mabel Todd, author of The Thinking Body and somatic educator explains this concept beautifully:

Hypermobility Without Tears

"The ability to improve a pattern of support and movement... Comes from the study and appreciation of the human body as a weight-bearing and weight-moving structure".

Now we are going to start at your feet. Your hands and feet have the most sensory receptors in the body – there is no better place to build sensory awareness.

EXERCISE – Open Your Sole

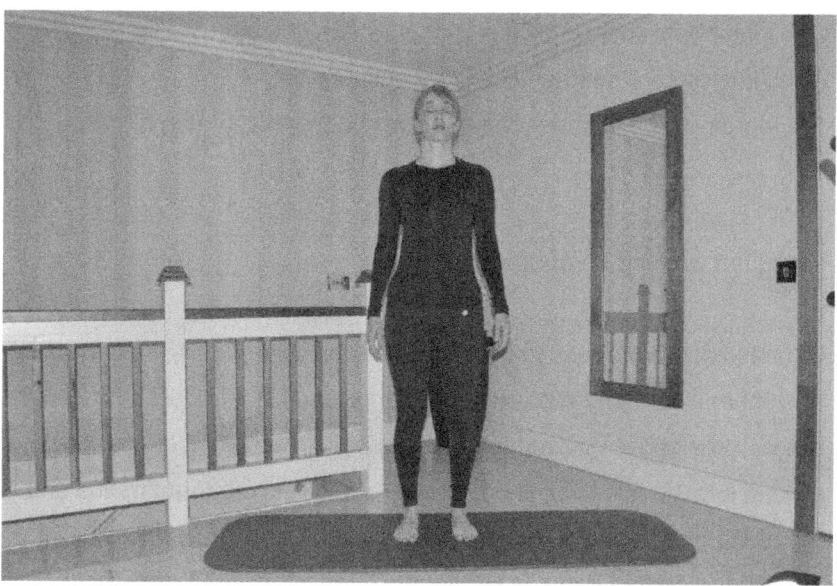

Chapter Three: Proprioception

Assume a standing position with bare feet – in whatever feels comfortable and pain free. Keep the knees soft and unlocked. This exercise will take a minimum of 5 minutes.

Close your eyes, if you are happy to. If you have a balance disorder, please keep your eyes open.

Notice how you feel, how you are standing, notice the thoughts coming in and out of your mind. Notice any tension in the feet, around the ankle or up the calf to the knee or lower back.

Send your attention down to your feet and observe them. How do they feel? What surface are you standing on? How does the surface feel under your feet? Where do you feel most of the weight in your feet? The front or the heels? Are you aware of your toes? Do they all touch the floor? Does one foot feel heavier than the other? Does one foot feel bigger?

Imagine the feet became so heavy, almost like you were wearing snowshoes, that you began to make a hole in the floor. What does the hole look like? Is one imprint deeper than the other? One foot bigger than the other? Are the feet straight on or turned out?

Allow your eyes to open and stand quietly for a moment.

Did you notice your feet for maybe the first time in years? Could you get a sense of your feet becoming heavier, more connected to the ground? We ideally want to create a sense of the weight of the legs and pelvis dropping down to the ground, with a large base of support to hold you. Imagine the feet are like the foundations of a house and the rest of your body are the walls, windows, chimney and roof that have to be able to feel secure on top of the foundations. When we allow this, we begin to feel the opposition of gravity – the upward thrust from the ground up.

When we respond to this upward thrust, this force can be used to allow the spine to release and open, giving us elongation. The spine will never open up to freedom, however, if the feet are not secure on the ground. This is why working the feet is so important to an integrated body.

I highly encourage you to practice standing with both feet firmly on the ground, as opposed to hanging off one hip, crossing the legs and all the other strange positions we may try to find comfort in. The more we practice, the easier and more comfortable it will become.

EXERCISE – Gentle Rock

From your standing posture above, let's try to distribute our weight across the ground beneath us to challenge our proprioception. Plus, it will give us a sense of when we are standing in equal balance on our feet.

Chapter Three: Proprioception

Begin to gently rock your body from left to right – but not enough to lift one foot off the floor. Try to experience a gentle increase in pressure on one foot and notice the other foot becomes lighter. Then repeat to the other side. Try not to side bend or twist your body as you do this – just move gently at the ankle joint.

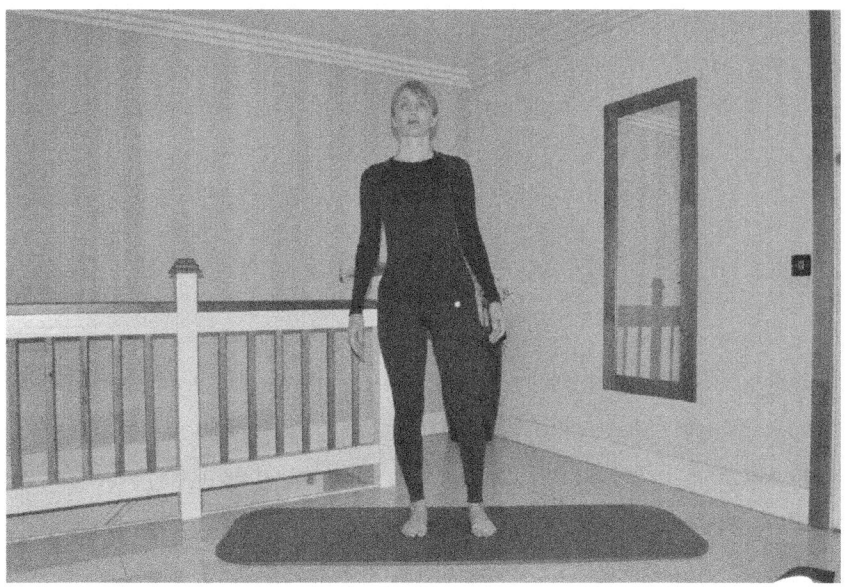

After you have got a good sense of this change in weight, try to move forwards and backwards in the same way. Keep the range small, without the heels or the toes coming off the floor. Notice how it feels when your body weight is too far forward or too far back. What sensations does this create?

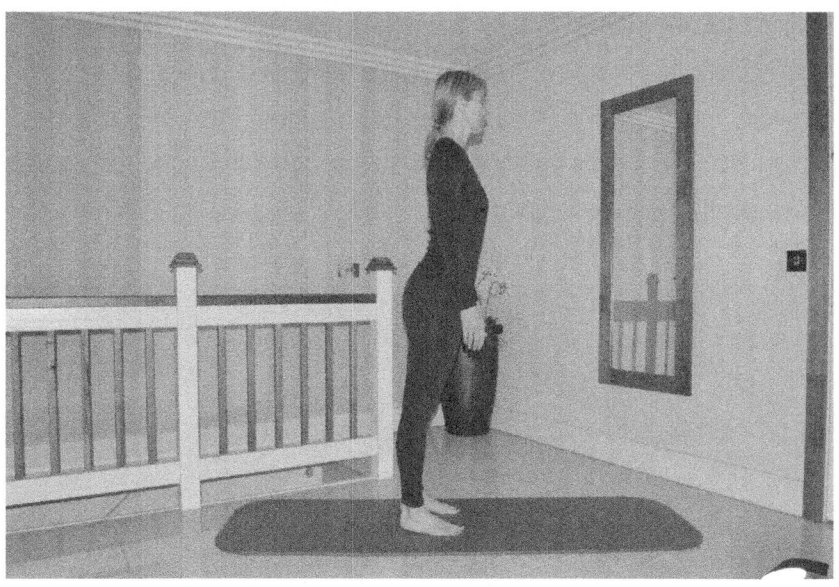

Finally, return to your centre place where both the feet feel equal, front and back and side to side. As you build and recognize this sensation, you will be able to find this in your everyday activities like standing in a queue, washing up, drinks parties or school events.

From there, we are going to challenge the feet and your awareness with a bridging pattern. The feet have a huge role in this movement – let's connect the relationship between the feet and the rest of the body.

Chapter Three: Proprioception

EXERCISE - Bridging

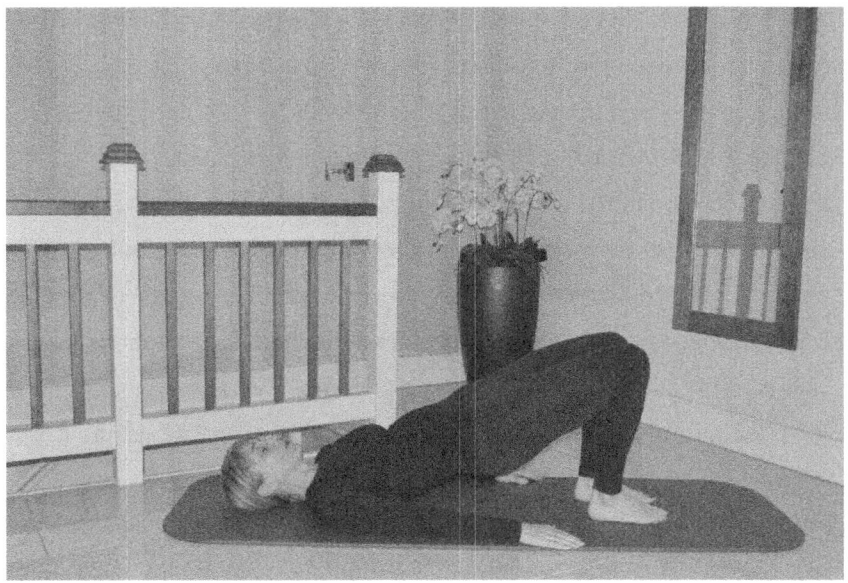

Assume a supine position and settle the body. Ensure your feet are not too far away from the pelvis, with the back of the heels in line with the sitting bones of the pelvis.

As you exhale, feel the weight sinking down through the feet into the floor. It is a sensation of almost making a hole in the floor because of the weight of the feet. As you feel the weight dropping down into your feet, allowing the feet to spread into the floor, can you feel as though the pelvis would like to float off the floor? Is there a sense of the pelvis feeling lighter than the legs and the feet?

Hypermobility Without Tears

The journey into the Bridge comes from the feet, from the weight dropping down into the feet so that the thigh bones are allowed to spiral out of the pelvis and travel away from the weightiness of the head. The aim is to remove tension from the front and back of the hips, removing any need to squeeze the buttocks. Allow the body to rest between the feet and the shoulders. Allow the front of your body to soften and drop into the back of your body. Can you settle into your feet so that your buttock muscles are not overworking? Are the feet balanced, left and right? Allow the front of the hips to open, but without being pushed – rather, breathe down into the thighs and create space with your breath. Do you feel the spine lengthen when it is not forced to? Create the space with your breath and the body will move into it.

Inhale at the top of the Bridge and begin the journey back down on the exhale. Travel down as you soften the roof of the mouth, the throat, the sternum, the ribcage and pelvis. The pelvis widens as it meets the floor, allowing the thigh bone to roll back into the hip socket. Are you able to meet the floor and find your settled position?

Pause and take as many breaths as you need to throughout each Bridge.

To build proprioception, we need to build control techniques. When we've been used to allowing our body to go into extraordinary ranges without our conscious awareness, it is essential we build consciousness. The following two exercises will help with this.

Chapter Three: Proprioception

EXERCISE – Supine Arm Roll

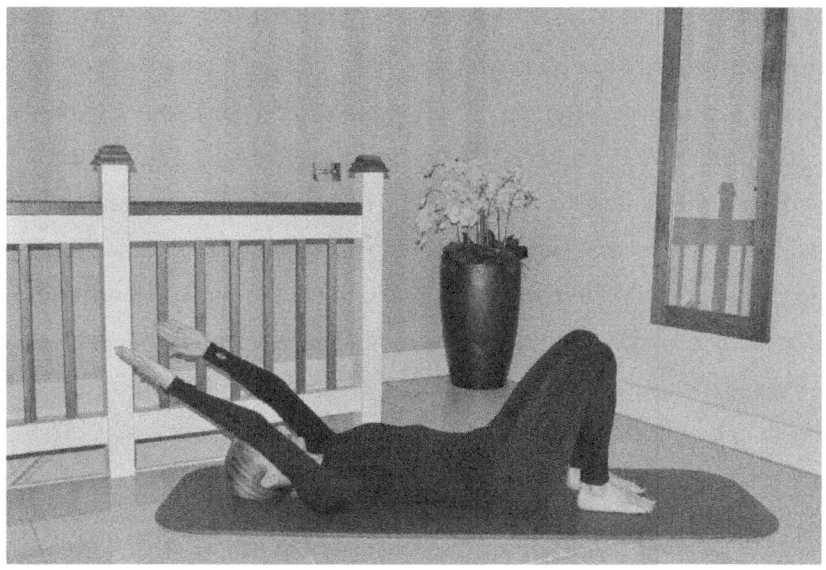

Assume a supine resting position, with your arms resting on the floor by your sides.

Find a weighty position of the feet, pelvis, ribs and head. Can you become aware of the back of your body touching the mat? Feel the weight of your shoulders resting on the mat. As you exhale, allow the shoulders to become heavier still. Can the upper arm bones become heavier than the forearm and hand? Can you draw attention to the back of the shoulders dropping down into the floor? As the upper arm bones continue to drop further down, allow the lower arm to float up off the floor until they start to rise above the head and pass over the head towards the wall behind you.

Be more focused on what is going on in the back of the body rather than what the arms are doing. Can you keep the back heavy into the mat as you move the arms? If you notice that your back has started to arch, it is time to stop the range there. The back needs to remain quiet and heavy as you move the arms. The back of the body includes the soles of your feet. If the arms drift in and out at this stage, do not worry. Be mindful as to what the back of your ribcage, back of pelvis and feet are doing at this moment. Are they still weighted and resting? Take a breath and notice if you can maintain the heaviness into the mat. The aim is not to take the arms to the floor, but rather notice how far you can really move without the back arching or feeling tense.

On an exhale, allow the arms to slowly float back down to the mat. Do not let them fall, but control them with the weight of your body.

Move only from the weightiness of the upper arm bones, so that the upper arm bone is able to roll in the shoulder socket. The top of the arm bone is round and it fits perfectly into the shoulder socket, allowing for ease of movement. Can you move without tension in the arms? Be aware of the arms moving from the back of your body so that there is little activity in the front of the shoulders. Allow the torso to rest completely through the whole process. We are trying not to pull the arms up off the floor, but rather roll them backwards in their socket.

Chapter Three: Proprioception

Pause at any time and let the body sink deeper with an extra out-breath.

It will of course be essential to discover our proprioceptive abilities when we are in non-weight bearing positions with the feet. Can we still explore and sense our body moving in space without the ground to support us as much?

Have a play with the following exercise for which you will need a medium strength stretch band.

EXERCISE – Exploring My Range

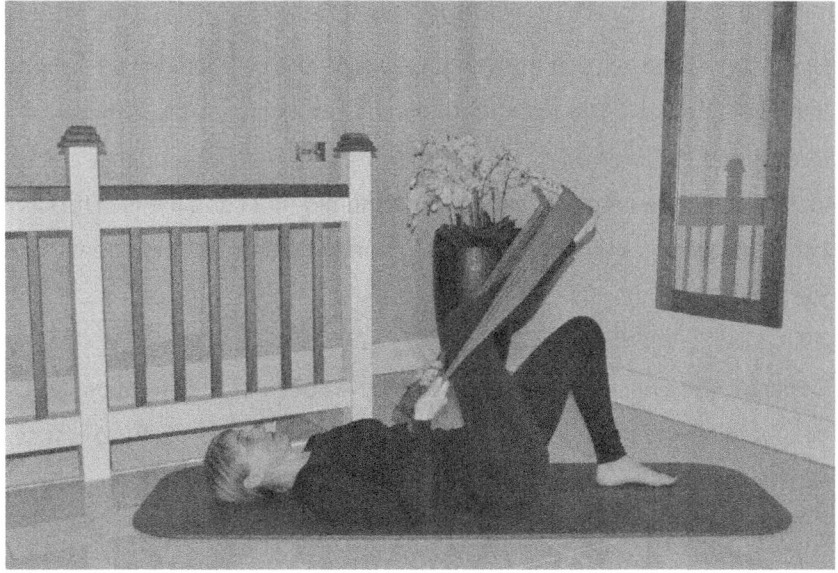

Hypermobility Without Tears

Lie on your back and place the band around one foot. Hold the band with both hands at the end. Start with the knee bent. Feel the weight of your thigh bone resting in the hip socket. Soften the hip, feel the weight of the pelvis under you. Slowly start to uncurl the leg, which will allow the leg to start to extend, but only allowing the leg to uncurl as a response to the weight of the thigh bone. Every time you exhale, allow the thigh bone to sink a little deeper into the hip socket. Every time it sinks, feel the hip socket becoming a little heavier. This will give a greater sense of connection and stability into the ground. Do not worry if the leg does not extend in a linear fashion – simply observe how you can extend your leg without pushing into the band with your foot. The movement starts because of the weight of the pelvis and the rolling action of the thigh bone in the pelvis. The out-breath will be quiet, slow and measured.

Slowly and gradually, let the leg get longer – the calf gets lighter as the thigh gets heavier. The back of the knee unfolds creating space here too, behind the knee joint. We want to feel space here as opposed to locking the knee joint and 'hanging' off the hip and knee joints. The low back is quiet and heavy into the mat. The shoulders are also heavy into the mat.

Continue this until the leg has unraveled. It does not matter if you cannot fully straighten the leg – that is not the objective of the exercise. We are avoiding pushing hard into the band – the fast pushing movement will destroy any sensitivity and could lead to a

Chapter Three: Proprioception

hyperextended knee joint. The key is slow and steady, using your breath to create the movement.

With this work we are seeking to build sensitivity. The proprioceptive awareness lies in the sensitivity to movements. If we fight and strive too hard, we risk not only to injure ourselves, but to miss the opportunity to build the much-needed connections in our body.

As Scaravelli stated "to be sensitive is to be alive". That is what we seek in our practice.

Hopefully this section has given you an insight into the role of proprioception in a hypermobile body. Remember, it is something that can be learnt and reprogrammed into your nervous system. Through building your sensory awareness and working with gravity, your proprioceptive abilities will naturally follow. Let's now move onto Stability.

Chapter Four: Stability
The Elusive Search

"It is doubtful that there exists a "core" group of trunk muscles that are recruited to operate independently of all other trunk muscles during daily activities... Muscle by muscle activation does not exist."
The myth of core stability, Dr Eyal Lederman, 2008

We learnt in the previous chapter the role of our fascia and our joints in proprioception and why it is important to build awareness of both. When we do this, we become more stable. I believe the locking of our joints is our unconscious way of seeking stability. The irony is, it makes us weaker and more vulnerable. We need a new, resilient strategy.

What do we mean by the term stability? If you perform a Google search for this term in relation to exercise, you will be inundated with results for 'core stability'. How many of you have been told you have a 'weak core' and that the only way out of pain is to strengthen your core? Invariably exercises then follow that involve the engagement of pelvic floor and transverse abdominal muscles – recruited by drawing up your pelvic floor and drawing your naval to your spine, thereby hollowing your

stomach. Let's just try that for one second. Go ahead and draw up your pelvic floor and suck in your stomach. Can you still breathe in the calm manner we learnt in Chapter One? Now imagine I asked you to keep that contraction for an hour while we do our exercise class. How does that make you feel? (You can let go now – that's enough of that.)
But hold on, surely that's something you're supposed to do always and forever – not just an hour a week in your exercise class? Surely if you have a weak core, you're going to have to keep those muscles engaged 24/7?

Quick answer – no. Please don't do that, ever. Remember we talked about the importance of breath and relaxation? How relaxed did you feel holding in your stomach? What I've seen time and time again are people who have been instructed to do this by therapists and teachers – Pilates being one of the worst offenders – and they are simply bound down by tension, guarding and the inability to move. And they are still in pain. The problem goes further with a hypermobile body – due to lack of proprioception, we will over recruit. We do not know the difference between a 10% recruitment and a 60% one. There's a chance we will seriously over-recruit, filling our body with bracing and tension. But when I teach these clients to unwind, release and move safely without that 'core' training, the pain dissipates. People start to have a sense of their own natural stability at play, without the need for bracing. Continue with the core strategy and you will have a pelvic girdle bound down and unable to move. That's a recipe for pain. We want a gliding, moveable pelvis – a central junction for the torso, arms and legs.

Chapter Four: Stability

You only need to look at children or animals moving if you want the answer. Do children get taught to draw in their abdominals before playing soccer or gym? Do dogs lift and tighten the pelvic floor before running for that ball? I don't think so. What we see is natural, free and fluid movements that they also enjoy.

The quote at the top of this chapter by Dr Lederman highlights that there is not one group of 'core' muscles. Everything is connected by this amazing network of connective tissue called fascia. When we are instructed to engage our pelvic floors and transverse abdominals, how do we know that these are the only muscles getting involved? They are so deep into the body you cannot feel them from external touch. What concerns me most about this approach to 'core stability' is stated in Lederman's paper when he quotes research of Brown et al in 2006:

"To specifically activate the core muscles during functional movement the individual would have to override natural patterns of trunk activation. This would be impractical, next to impossible and potentially dangerous."

We are trying to create fluid, natural and pain-free movements. Why would we attempt to disrupt this natural ability in the body by forcing it to work in this way? On top of this, Lederman also states that if you are taught to do these contractions lying on your back, there is no guarantee this will even translate to a functional movement like standing, running, lifting and so on. We put a great deal of stress and strain on the body for apparent little benefit. We must have a more efficient, pain-free solution available to us. But if bracing and fixing is not the answer to our stability, what is? The answer is gravity. It is your movement's best friend. It makes movement easier, freer and improves much-needed proprioception. Stability comes from the feedback the body receives through proprioception and contact with the ground – whether this be lying down, standing, sitting or in a quadruped position. It is the role of the sensory receptors in the connective tissue to inform your brain.

The research for my Integral Movement Method (IMM) was greatly inspired by the work of yogi Vanda Scaravelli. She talks of a 'revolution' where 'the pushing and pulling has come to an end' (Scaravelli 1991). I found this way of thought was not common in the Pilates teachings. I brought this way of moving into my method. I particularly like her quote "the muscles must not be activated through tension or effort but only through the much more powerful wave of extension, which is produced by gravity and breathing". She refers to this force as an 'anti-gravity reflex'. I call this 'ground force' – that almost pushes us away from the ground in response to gravitational pull. Newton's Third Law of Motion states that "for every action there is an equal and opposite reaction".

Let's look at some practical movements to help foster our understanding of the body's natural stability.

Chapter Four: Stability

EXERCISE – Supine Hip Roll

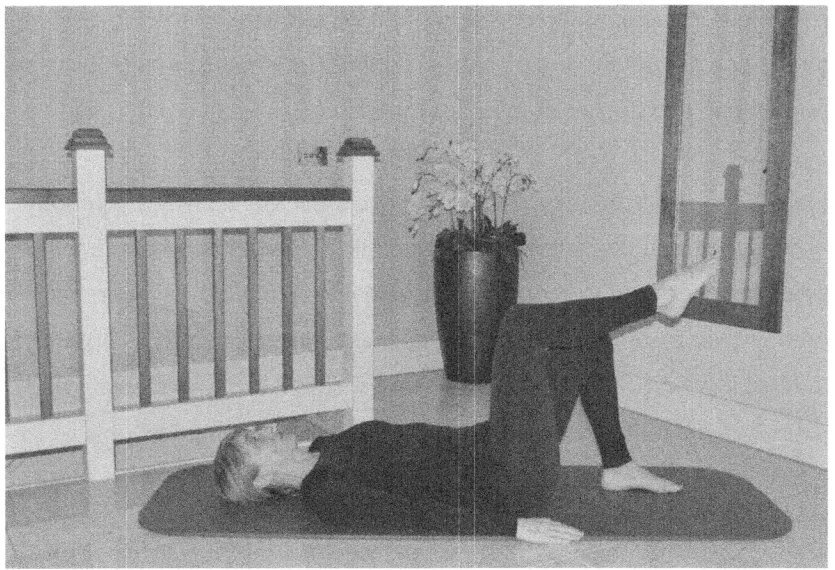

Assume a supine position and establish a sense of heaviness into the floor.

Draw attention to the weightiness of the pelvis. The movement here will be facilitated by the out-breath, so take a full deep inhale. As you exhale, feel the pelvis getting weightier. On the following exhale, when you feel the pelvis is at its heaviest, get a sense of one of your legs becoming lighter. So as the torso becomes heavier, can you allow one leg to become lighter? As we sink down into the mat, we can allow the thigh bone to roll into the socket. Again, the top of the thigh bone is round and it rolls into the hip socket freely if allowed. We do not need to lift the leg up off the floor, but rather allow a rolling action in towards the body. The bones are round, the pelvis is round – they are designed to roll together. Look for a sensation of heaviness around the top of the thigh bone so that the knee can feel lighter. Can the tissue of your thigh remain soft and tension-free?

Ideally, the aim is to keep all the body weight into the back of the body, allowing the body to settle so that it can find a sense of lightness to the limb that is moving. Without sensing heaviness in the torso, there is a greater chance of the lumbar or thoracic spine arching or tensing when the limbs are moving. The torso wants to remain quiet and lengthened, almost undisturbed by the movement of the surrounding limbs.

Hold the position for one breath and, on an exhale, slowly lower the leg down with control. Try not to allow gravity to drop the leg quickly to the floor. Let the leg settle once it meets the floor.

Chapter Four: Stability

EXERCISE – Double Supine Hip Roll

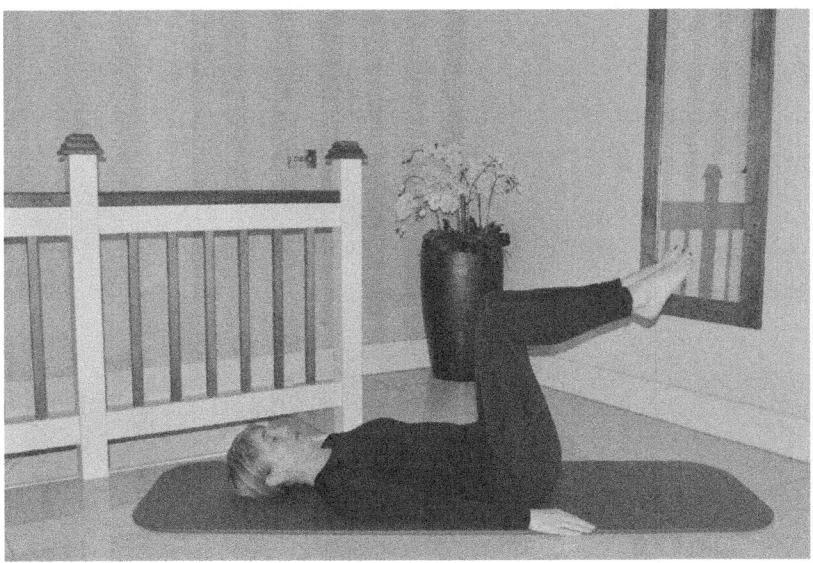

Once you have become familiar and confident with a Supine Hip Roll, the progression would be to lift the second leg up off the floor. Before we attempt this, we must ensure that there is no lumbar arch of the spine when lifting just one leg. If you are able to maintain a heavy pelvis without movement, feel free to explore the double leg version.

Repeat the format for the single leg version. Once the first leg is in the air, take another inhale. As you exhale, allow the pelvis to sink further into the mat. When you are at your heaviest point (probably when you are almost out of air), you can allow the second leg to float off the floor to join the first one. The pelvis and spine remain heavy and unchanged by this action.

Return the legs to the floor one at a time, using your exhale to help facilitate the movement. Again, the lumbar spine should not arch as you lower the leg down.

EXERCISE – Quadruped Organisation

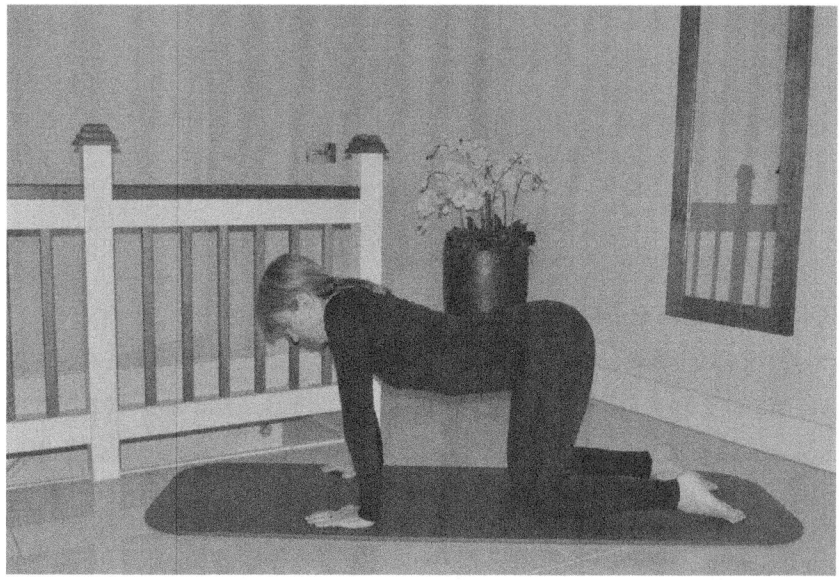

This position can be particularly challenging for someone with hypermobility for many reasons. The temptation to sink into the lower

Chapter Four: Stability

back and allow the upper spine to collapse between the shoulders is great. This inevitably comes with the hyperextension of the elbow and poor head position. But with the use of gravity, as we have been exploring in this book, we can learn how to organize ourselves here too. The knees, shins, front of foot and sole of hands are now the only contact points we have with the floor. Our aim is to establish a sense of weightiness into these points. As we have discovered, the more weight that is put into the floor, the lighter and freer the spine becomes. Therefore, allow the weight to fall through the hands and lower limbs, giving the spine a sense of drawing away from the mat. Can you move your pelvis forward and backwards without disturbing your spine? If so, you will be able to then establish your resting pelvis in this position – not too far forward so that the spine is rounded and not too far back causing the back to arch.

In order to understand where the head should be in space (without any feedback now from the floor or support), we have to use our contact points. The more you have awareness of the hands into the floor, the more the head can float away from the ground. Top tip – ears always point forwards, not up or down. See if you can hold this position comfortably for two to three breaths.

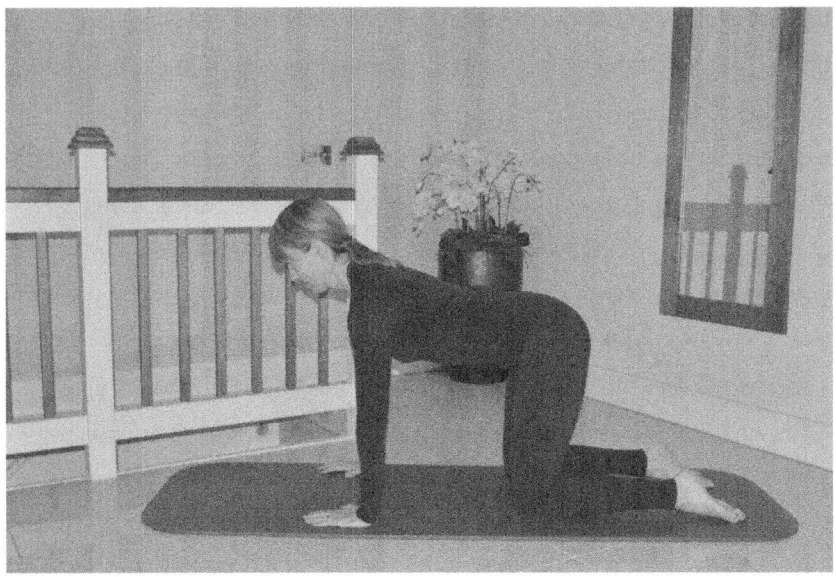

EXERCISE – Quadruped Hip Hinge

Once we have established an organised quadruped position, we can challenge it with movement.

Once comfortable, allow the front of your hips to soften, almost as though you wanted to create a big crease in the front of your trousers. Allow the body to sink backwards into this crease, but at the same time maintaining the spine long. The spine ideally does not round or arch but maintains a quiet resting place as you allow the rotation of the hip bone in the hip socket.

As you move backwards, can you get a sense of the breastbone sliding forwards? Can the shoulders and arms rest tension-free? There is no

Chapter Four: Stability

pushing with the arms to move backwards, but rather softening into the hip. Can you breathe easily in this position? If you have any knee pain or prior injury – please keep the range of knee flexion to a position that is comfortable.

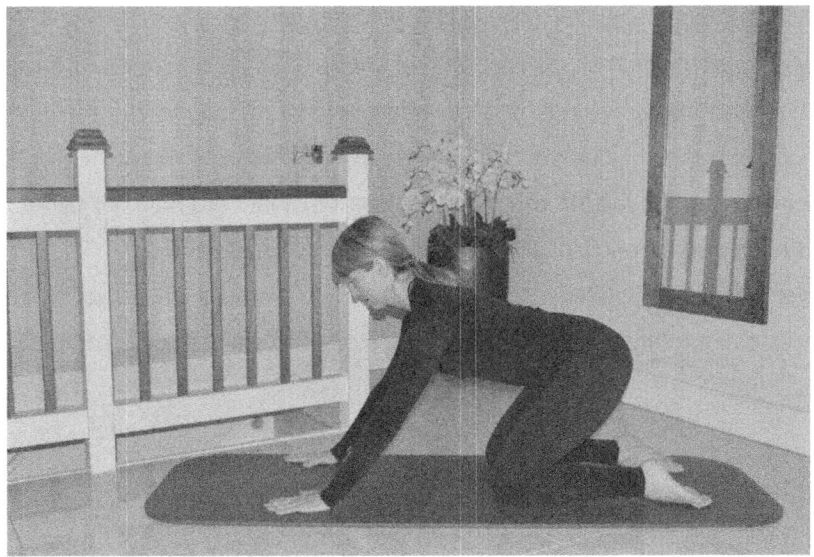

When you are ready to return, use an exhale to drop weight further down into the shins and hands and draw the body forward and up at the same time.

EXERCISE – Quadruped Shoulder Stability with Small Ball

I love this exercise for challenging our proprioception and balance whilst in a quadruped position. Assume a well-organized position and place a small ball under one hand. Try not to collapse into the ball but rather rest your hand lightly on the ball. As you exhale, can you roll the ball away from you? There will be several things to look out for: check the supporting elbow has not hyperextended; check the supporting shoulder has not collapsed; check the lumbar spine has not arched or rounded. As you roll the ball away, try not to fall into the ball, but rather maintain your strong position with shoulders square to the floor. The objective is not to roll the ball out too far but to maintain the quadruped organization comfortably. When ready, exhale to roll the ball back to you.

Chapter Four: Stability

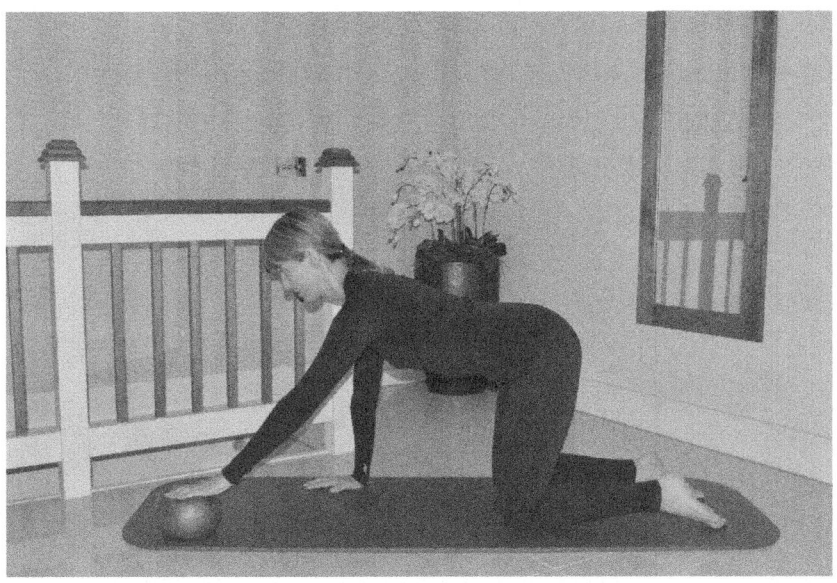

A discussion on stability would not be complete without covering the topic of stretching. It is the number one question I get asked by the hypermobile community – should I be stretching and is it safe? This is a hot topic with differing views. In my experience, static stretching is not beneficial for a hypermobility body for a number of reasons.
Firstly, static stretching gives the opportunity for 'hanging' in the joints. This is not at all beneficial for the joint or surrounding connective tissue.

You notice on photo a) that I am closer to the floor but there is no support being offered by the ground – remember how important working with gravity is and the ability to receive the ground force into the body. I am literally hanging off of my lumbar spine and hamstrings. This is not going to help build the tonality that we need for strong resilient connective tissue. The joints are in a vulnerable position for damage. In photo b), I am not as close to the floor but there is work being done. I use my feet to give me an upward thrust from the ground. Therefore, when we make contact with the ground there is an opposite force exerted from the ground. There is a balance of the forces.

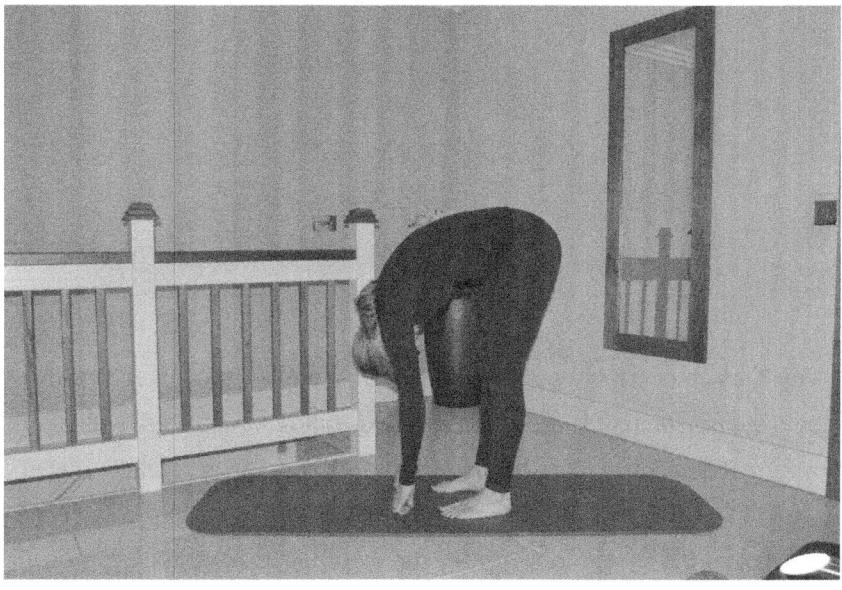

Photo a) demonstrates 'hanging' in the joints – incorrect posture.

Chapter Four: Stability

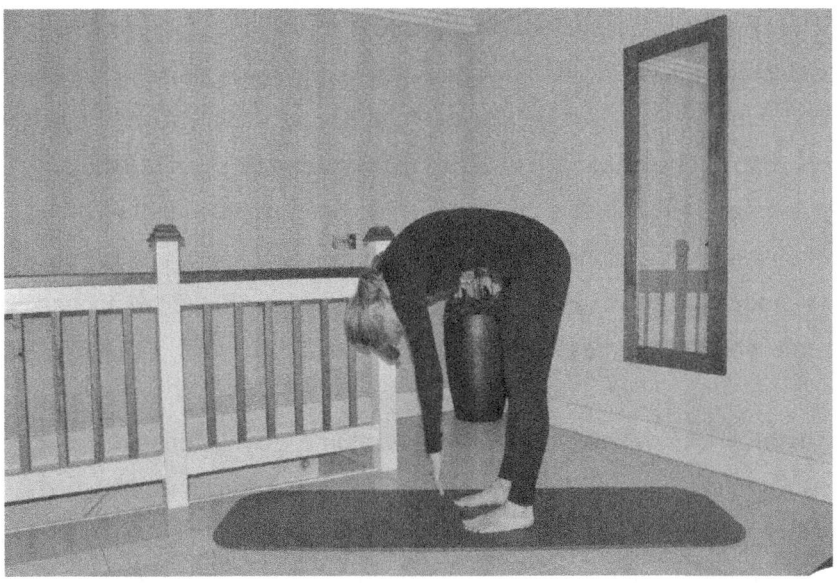

Photo b) demonstrates a supported position with muscle activation – correct posture.

Secondly, static stretching may feel great at the time but often not so great the following day. Hypermobile bodies are often stiff in some areas but loose in others. The tight areas are tight for a very good reason. They are desperately trying to stabilise and hold together your whole structure. Muscles may also become tight because they are pulling on unstable joints that do not respond with the appropriate amount of stiffness.

Hypermobility Without Tears

If you continue to stretch these tight areas to end of range, you risk taking away the very thing that gave your brain some sense of security and stability – however imbalanced that may be. The hypermobile body will grab at anything it can to find stability – even muscles like the diaphragm. I'm including myself here too, but a common strategy is often to use the diaphragm – your key muscle for breathing – to hold the body up. I see a lot of rib gripping and tension around the ribcage area, which of course has implications for breathing well.

Thirdly, we know that proprioception is often a lacking sense as explored in Chapter Three. This means we could stretch way beyond a healthy range without even realizing. We are stretching that already compromised connective tissue, which by the nature of this condition already has a hard time with elasticity. Joints will also tend to stretch before the tight fascia or muscle – potentially leading to injury. We learnt in the previous chapter than the fascia is filled with sensory receptors – that is what is going to hurt when you stretch too much. We will talk more about the importance of creating an elastic body in the Posture chapter.

I'm not a great fan therefore of stretching for stretching's sake. I do however believe we need to encourage movement within those tight areas. We do need to stretch these muscles, but in a way that is safe and appropriate for a hypermobile body. It is not healthy or functional to have restrictions in the body. What we seek is a fluid body that has the ability of the tissue to glide one layer on top of the other with control.

Chapter Four: Stability

Our muscles are dense – there are several layers beneath the skin. For pain-free movement, each layer needs to be able to glide easily on the one above and / or below. That's a big ask especially if we have not been moving regularly through injury, pain or fear.

I promote this gliding and freedom with controlled dynamic stretching. This means we learn to move in and out of a stretch – without holding it – but we still experience the sensation of a stretch. Instead of just stretching the tissue, though, we build elasticity. With dynamic stretching you are not going to have the chance to go to end of range, thereby preventing strain and injury. Dynamic stretching improves control and proprioception when executed correctly. In the book Fascia in Sport and Movement (2015), Schliep states that long-term and regular use of dynamic stretching can positively influence the architecture of the connective tissue in that it becomes more elastic.

Let's take a look at a couple of my favorite dynamic stretches.

EXERCISE – CAT with Hip Softener

The CAT is a familiar exercise, yet it can often be overdone with a hypermobile body. In our desire to stretch out those tight upper back muscles, we could be tempted to push into our arms. This will cause an over-flexion of the thoracic spine and a flattening of the lumbar curve (see photo a). Ideally, the CAT should be used to create an even distribution of the forces going through the spine in flexion. If you see the second picture (photo b), the curve of the spine looks more even and my arms are visibly softer. Can we therefore create the CAT position first without the hyperextension in the joints? Try to move in and out of CAT for a few times without pushing.

Chapter Four: Stability

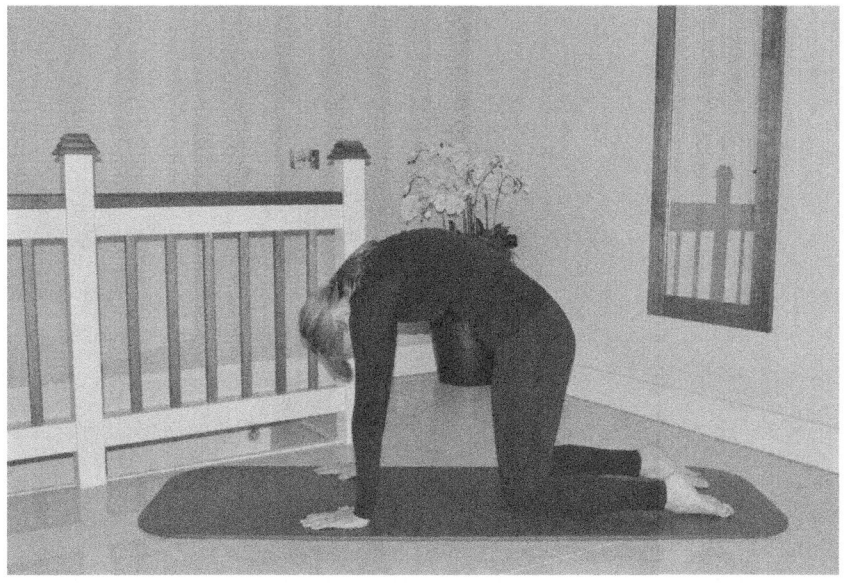

Photo a) demonstrates pushing into the arms and upper back to 'feel' a stretch – poor posture.

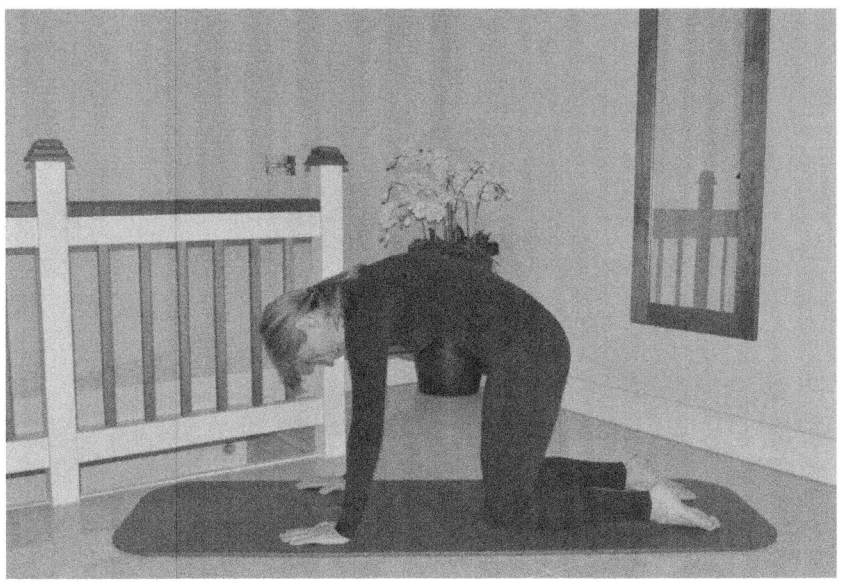

Photo b) demonstrates a softer spinal curve without hyperextension in the joints – good posture.

Once familiar with the pattern, add in the hip softener from the previous exercise. Keep the CAT shape and soften the front of the hips so that the body travels backwards. This usually results in a stretch through the back of the body. With dynamic stretching, we do not stay and hold the position, but we move in and out of this stretch smoothly and slowly to 'tease' the fascia into letting go. It's important to breathe into the back of the ribs here – as we explored in our prone breathing exercise earlier.

Chapter Four: Stability

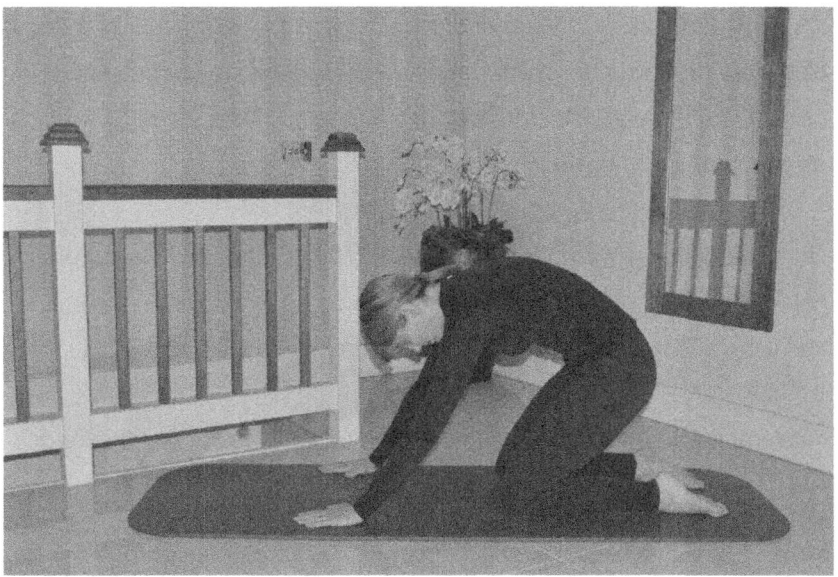

EXERCISE – Forward Roll

Establish a standing posture with equal balance between the feet. Find your feet and allow them to spread into the floor. This exercise can be practiced against a wall too to begin with – the pelvis stays supported against a wall while you roll down.

Feel you are drawn down by the weight of your legs. As the legs get heavier, allow the head to nod and begin to slowly roll forward through the spine on an exhale. We are aiming not to collapse into the joints. Try to find the spine lifting up and out of the pelvis into the roll forward. The spine will lengthen away from the heavy draw of the legs.

Hypermobility Without Tears

As we flex the spine forward and down, notice the abdominal wall draws backwards towards the spine. Ideally, we keep the weight balanced through both feet without hinging onto the heels. Take as many breaths as you need to go down.

On the way down allow the knees to bend if you need to. It is important not to allow the knees to hyperextend here – better to soften the knees and allow a bend.

Inhale at the bottom and send the breath up into the back of the lungs.

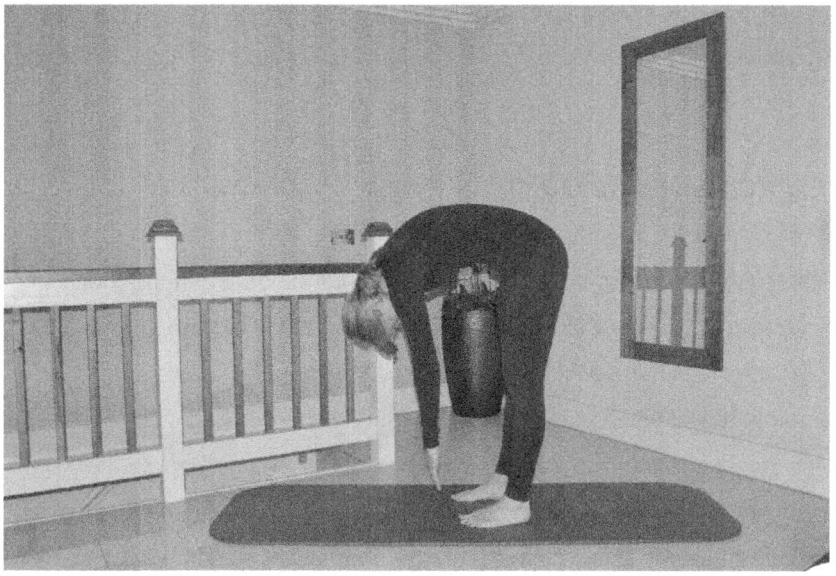

As you exhale, stand down into your feet. Feel the feet dropping down into the floor. Notice the response again of the abdominal wall, as it

Chapter Four: Stability

draws up and back into the body. Follow that motion of drawing up and back as you roll back upright re-establishing a standing posture. Can you go down to come up?

Tip: your legs should be working as your roll up, allowing the spine to unravel freely.

Remember – it is important not to 'hang' in this posture. Keep the legs working at all times but this will allow an opening of the backline of the body. It is a good way to allow the hamstrings to lengthen and contract in a healthy way.

Hypermobility Without Tears

EXERCISE – Side Lying Arm Roll

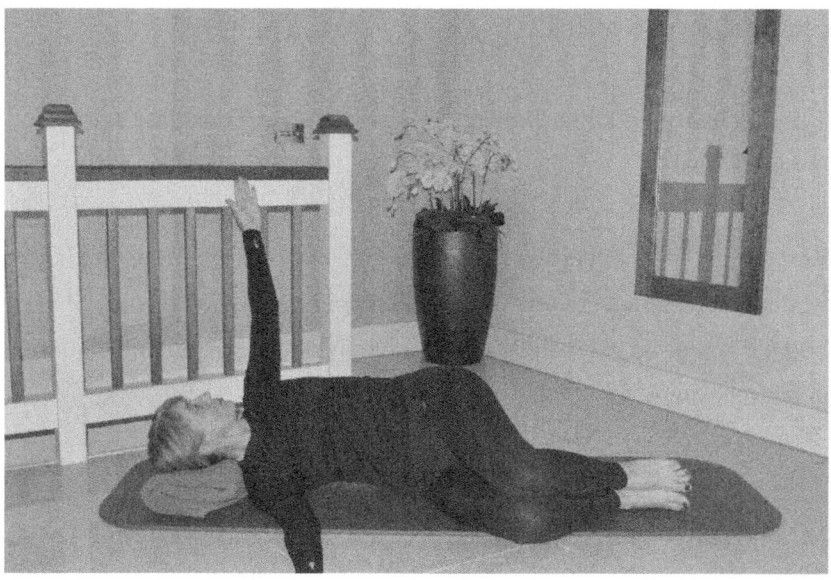

The front of the chest can be an area of tightness. This exercise allows us to open up the front body with full support from the floor. Side-lying challenges our awareness further as we have a narrow part of the body in contact with the mat. This is a comfortable way to enhance rotational movement of the spine. For ideal head and neck alignment, please use a rolled-up towel or head cushion to support the head.

Assume a side-lying position with knees bent – as though you were seated on a chair. Place your arms together in front of the body. Establish the sense of heaviness into the points of contact with the

Chapter Four: Stability

floor. Try to maintain a lengthened waist so that the waist is not collapsed into the floor.

As you exhale, feel the weight of the top shoulder blade drawing down to your mid back. As with the Supine Arm Rolls, can you get a sense of the upper arm bone being heavier than the forearm, so that the upper arm is able to roll down into the shoulder socket, enabling it to then roll up until the finger tips point at the ceiling? Keep looking at the hand as your neck allows. Do not strain the neck to see the arm.

Once the fingertips are pointing up at the ceiling, take a further exhale and begin to roll the ribs away from the knees – rotating the spine and maintaining the gaze on the hand. Try to keep the arm still and settled in the shoulder socket. Feel the weight of the legs and the other arm resting on the floor. Do not let the moving arm fall to the floor behind you – keep it connected into the back of the body.

Tip: if you cannot see the inside length of your arm, you have gone too far. There may be a sensation of stretching at the front of the chest in the pectoral area now.

Inhale into the top ribs and feel the ribcage expand. Exhale, holding the position to see if that facilitates any further rotation of the spine.

Hypermobility Without Tears

When you are ready to return, use the exhale to roll the ribs, carrying the arm in its socket back to face the front. Allow the arm to float back down and rest on top.

You may notice one side of the body feels different to the other.

Before we close this chapter, this is an appropriate place to mention range of movement. We know that hypermobile bodies can have the ability to move into ranges that other people may struggle to achieve. The strategy I always use with my clients to begin with is introducing a reduced range of movement. They hate it because it is so much harder trying to control the body than allowing it to 'hang out' at end of range. But this is essential to the IMM and our health – we will never build the sensitivity until we experience what a 'normal' range of movement feels like. The nervous system will never learn a new pattern if the body is allowed to continue to end range movement. Through controlled, shorter range movement the body pays attention. It notices if the alignment changes, if the spine lifts away from the mat. In the photo below, the aim is not to achieve a big range of arm movement, but rather control the weight of the spine into the floor. My range is determined by my ability to control the spine.

Chapter Four: Stability

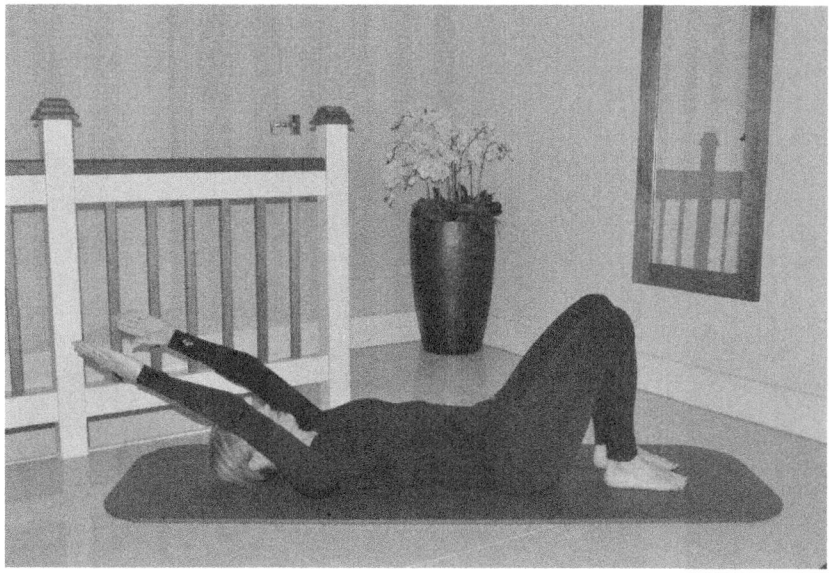

Once we have established an understanding, ranges can be increased. We do not want to lose freedom of movement, but we have to know how to control it, how to work with it safely and effectively. By following the IMM you will have a strong body that can move freely, with the support and cooperation of the whole system.

We will explore the whole body system in greater depth in the following chapter – Balance.

Chapter Five: Balance
The Daily Challenge

"When the foot hits the ground, a whole body reaction occurs"
Gary Ward, Author – What The Foot, 2013

Balance is essential for everyday life. The act of walking is itself a balancing act as we transfer body weight from one foot to another. If we are not comfortable in standing balance work, we may create fear around walking and mobility. If you have been a wheelchair or walking aid user, it is going to be normal to be anxious around balance work. The good news is that balance can be taught. If you have been working through the book and completing the exercises as you go, you will already have been building your sensory awareness. Sensory awareness is going to be a key ingredient for balance, together with the understanding of the ground force at play. Without this, balance is always going to be a challenge. The IMM takes you on a progressive, structured journey – introducing you to each element in the appropriate order. By following the steps laid out, you will achieve the greatest success.

Hypermobility Without Tears

When working with clients I always turn my attention to their feet pretty quickly into the assessment process. We touched on the role of the feet in Chapter Three. When we come to training balance, I am looking for alignment of the foot, ankle and lower limb, together with a degree of mobility and stability. These factors are going to create positive or negative impacts in your body further up the chain – such as hip pain, low back pain and even shoulder pain. With a hypermobile body, flat feet or collapsed arches are common. The muscles in the feet can become deconditioned in the same way as any other muscle would in the body. The foot is made up of 26 bones, 33 joints and more than 100 muscles, ligaments and tendons. That gives us great potential for movement – in many cases too much. Sprained ankles and ligaments can be a regular occurrence for a hyper mobile body. What we need to do therefore is to find a way to give the foot structure the support and strength it needs, whilst maintaining a mobile foot. The design of the foot tells us it is meant to move. It would not have these many joints if it were supposed to be static, rigid and underutilized. Through my program, I have introduced wheelchair users to the amazing ability of their feet to recover and become strong, functioning pieces of equipment.

The second important aspect of the foot is that its positioning is going to impact the alignment of the whole of the body. If a foot is over pronated – with flat feet that do not respond to the forces put onto it (i.e. it allows the foot to collapse into the ground taking the rest of the limb with it) –

Chapter Five: Balance

the rest of the body will follow this line of force. It brings us right back to the issue of how we respond to gravity and the ground force.

With a pronated foot, the lower limb, knee and thigh bone tend to role inwards towards the midline of the body. This will impact the position of the pelvis, lower back and so on up the chain to the head. The correct positioning of the foot is therefore paramount to the organisation of the whole body. Things can be mixed too – some people have two pronated feet but some only have one. The other foot may be well aligned. You then have different tensions running through the body.

Either way it can be a recipe for pain. Walking can result in pain and not just foot pain. Due to the impact on the whole body, the pain could travel anywhere up the chain. If there is pain on walking, the brain could make the decision to avoid the action that is painful. We could become more immobile as a result.

The problem anyone has with this strategy is the pain / exercise cycle. It applies to everyone but seems to impact hypermobile bodies to a greater degree due to the already lax connective tissue.

Hypermobility Without Tears

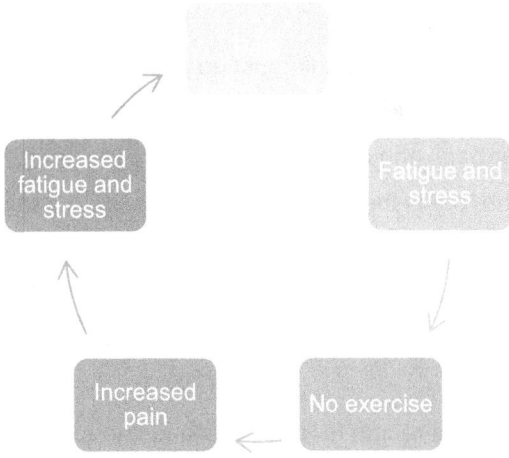

Pain causes stress and fatigue. If you've been in pain for a long period of time, it is a natural response to be stressed about that. Coping with pain is exhausting too, so we have this relationship between pain, stress and fatigue. Understandably, we are reluctant to exercise at this point for a variety of reasons: we feel tired; we are worried that the exercise will make the pain worse; we have fear around exercise itself. There may even be disbelief that exercise can in fact help anyway – many of us have been through poor past exercise experiences that have made us feel worse. So, we leave it hoping that rest will make the pain and stress go away. But it is hard to rest properly when you are in pain, so that often does not work out well. For the majority of hypermobile bodies leaving it without exercise makes things worse

Chapter Five: Balance

because the longer we go without movement, the more deconditioned our bodies become. Deconditioned tissue causes further pain because it has to work even harder now to function, to hold us together or do our daily activities. On top of this deconditioned tissue, it leads to more stress and fatigue as we can probably sense ourselves spiraling deeper into this cycle. It is a vicious cycle.

Ideally, we need to introduce small amount of movement to break this vicious pain cycle. I am not saying this will be easy and it may not be the preferred first choice of action, but it is essential for the road to recovery. We have to move, but we have to move appropriately, and we have to move well. Throwing ourselves wholeheartedly into the wrong approach is not going to give a positive movement experience. I am therefore definitely not recommending we go and workout at the gym 7 days a week whether we are exhausted or not. But I am saying that small, little-and-often exercise and movement therapy is going to help. We start slow, no pressure, no expectations. We rest when we need to rest, but we do need to build a habit of movement into our lives. That's where the IMM – a no pain, no strain exercise program – can really help. It's how I rehabbed myself and it is how I now work with all my hypermobile and EDS clients.

"I'm not sure if I can express the extent of my gratitude in words. Just that one session has changed my life with a view of complete recovery. After maybe a couple of hours after the session those hot spots on my

Hypermobility Without Tears

back completely melted off, I'm amazed and so grateful, thank you so much".
Ashley, hypermobile client

Let's get started at the ground up.

We need to get to know our feet first. Maybe a podiatrist has told you that you have flat feet. You may have orthotics to correct this. It would be great to train the muscles of the feet and lower legs to build strength and resilience. It is possible to rebuild the arches of the feet. I've done it many times with clients. Once we have an arch, we have a structure that is responsive to the ground and the forces put through it in actions like walking, running and standing.

Just think about the famous Roman arches. When they crumble, the structure above them starts to fall about too. The arch is the foundation on which everything else rests. It is therefore essential that we train and exercise the muscles of our feet just like we would any other muscle. We need to build a sense of the movement in the feet and their ability to offer a solid base of support and stability. Unless you feel supported when you stand, the rest of the body is forced to 'hang on' just to operate. You could end up working harder than you need to just to get around and cause yourself additional pain in the process. You will also use more vital energy, leading to fatigue.

Chapter Five: Balance

Remove your shoes and socks and stand for a moment. Take a look at your feet or, even better, have someone take a photo of them for you. What do your feet look like? Does the structure look like it is rolling inwards? Where is the pressure in your feet? Inside edges, front of foot, heels? Is your big toe lifted up or able to rest on the ground? Any bunions, hard skin areas, corns? Sit down and take a feel around your feet. Does one foot have more hard skin than the other? These are all little signals that tell you how you are using your feet, how much force you are putting through each foot and on what part of the foot.

For a balanced body, we would like to see an evenness of weight through both feet. In an ideal world, there would be the same force going through both feet. Both feet would have a 'neutral' alignment in standing – but this neutral alignment would change dynamically with movement. It is ok to move the feet into pronation; in fact, it is an essential part of the gait cycle. Pronating the foot is what prepares the foot to propel you forward in motion. The problem occurs when the feet have collapsed into over-pronation and are not responsive enough to return back through supination. The muscles and connective tissue in the feet are deconditioned and have lost the all-important elasticity to move your forward. We therefore need to use more effort and strain to 'pick up the leg' to walk, as opposed to an elastic recoil that we all have. We simply need to train this and start to use our natural gait patterns. This movement issue can be fairly common in hypermobility. As it is about the tone of the muscle, it means that we can train this.

Hypermobility Without Tears

The body is really happy when there is equal balance through both feet. If we are able to retrain ourselves to find an equal 50% split of weight between both legs and feet, our body is immediately going to start to find a new relationship with the ground.

Try it now – stand up and notice if you have an equal distribution through the feet. This is a very important question – it tells us a great deal about how you may be operating on a daily basis. If for example, you felt you had 70% of your body weight on one foot and only 30% on the other you are favoring one side of your body over the other. This will be reflected in all of your daily movements, like walking. If one side of your body is having to work 20% harder, this is potentially going to cause us pain and discomfort – anywhere in the body. So having the ability to find balance evenly across both feet is going to be essential for our whole body health. I encourage you to gently explore this exercise to see if you can achieve a 50/50 split without causing too much discomfort. It will take time especially if you had a big difference to begin with so please do not be disheartened. Take a few moments every day to stand and notice your feet.

The following series of short movements will really help you connect with your feet, improve mobility and strength of the whole lower leg.

Chapter Five: Balance

EXERCISE – Big Toe Lift

Whilst maintaining your even balance in your feet, can you lift your big toe up – without lifting any of the other toes? This will start to build strength in the muscle supporting the big toe joint.

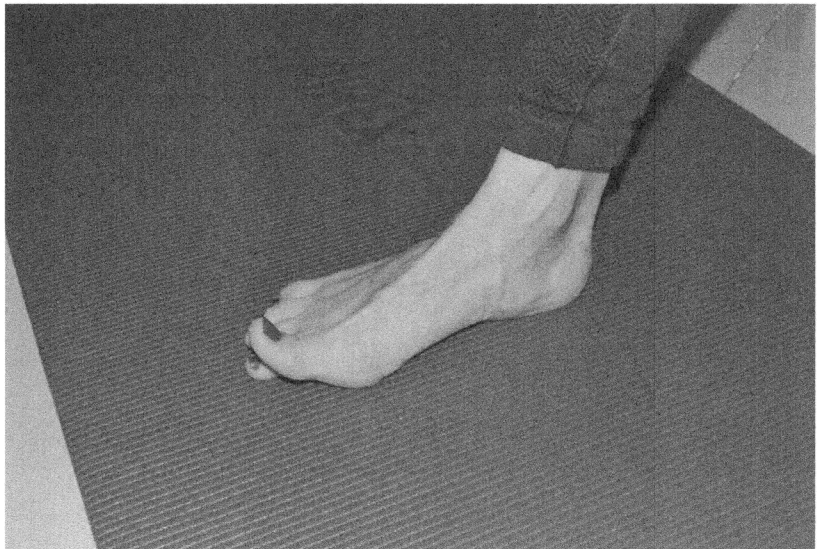

EXERCISE – Four Toe Lift

Can you now lift the other four toes – leaving the big toe on the ground?

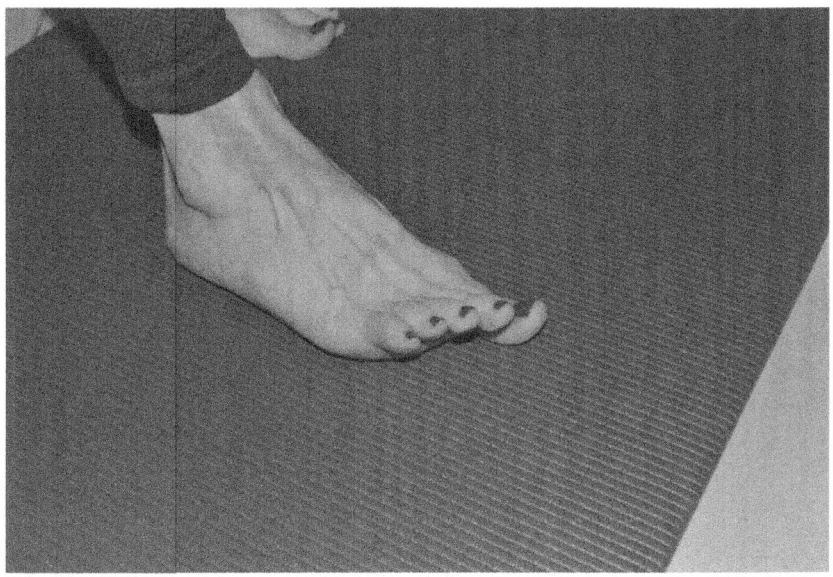

EXERCISE – Ankle Rotations

Whilst sitting, keep the knee stable and try to rotate the ankle in both directions. It is tempting to over recruit the toes, so try to keep these quiet and focus on the ankle mobility.

Chapter Five: Balance

EXERCISE – Heel Raises with Ball

This is a great move to build all important strength in the front of the foot. I find the tennis ball is particularly helpful if you are hypermobile as it gives extra feedback. Place a tennis ball just below the ankle bones and hold is firmly but do not squeeze it hard. Hold onto a chair initially for balance (but eventually we would like to do this without holding on). As you exhale, feel the pressure increase in the front of the foot. As the front foot gets heavier, allow the heels to rise up off the floor. Keep hold of the tennis ball as you do this. Inhale at the top and exhale to slowly lower the heels to the floor.

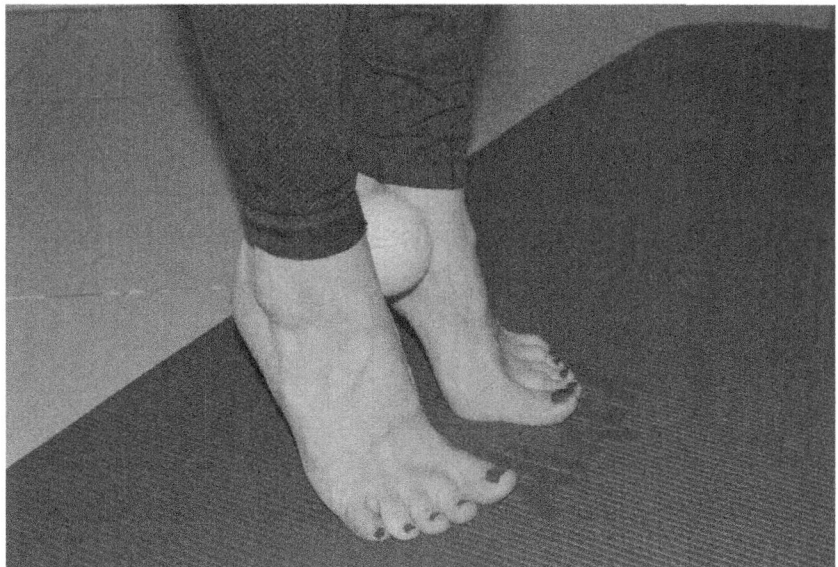

EXERCISE – Standing Hip Softener

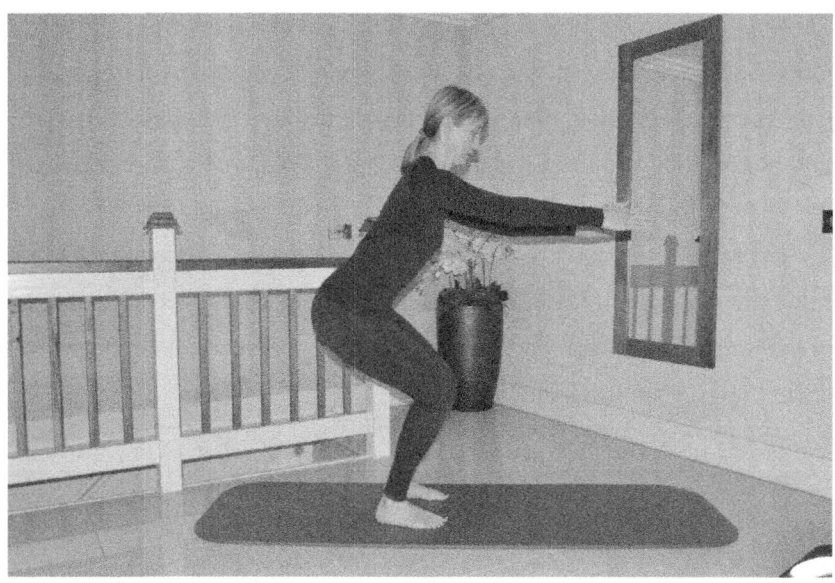

Establish your standing posture with equal weight on both feet. Avoid extreme knee flexion if you experience knee pain. This should feel comfortable throughout the body. Aim to keep the spine lengthened, breastbone moving away from the pelvis.

Rather than approaching this as a squat and pressing down into the joints, allow the hips to soften backwards, which causes the knees to fall forward. The movement is initiated at the hip joint – as though you were about to sit on a chair. As you soften backwards, the arms can float forwards with the shoulders resting on the ribcage. Try to establish

Chapter Five: Balance

a sense of widening of the sitting bones and the front of the hips simultaneously. Keep awareness of the feet. As we come into our Hip Softener position, the feet are going to need to spread out more into the floor.

To stand up, rather than pulling yourself up using your spinal muscles, send the feet down into the ground. Again, can you go down to go up? As the legs work more, the spine finds a lightness and lengthens back up into standing.

EXERCISE – Side-lying Leg Roll

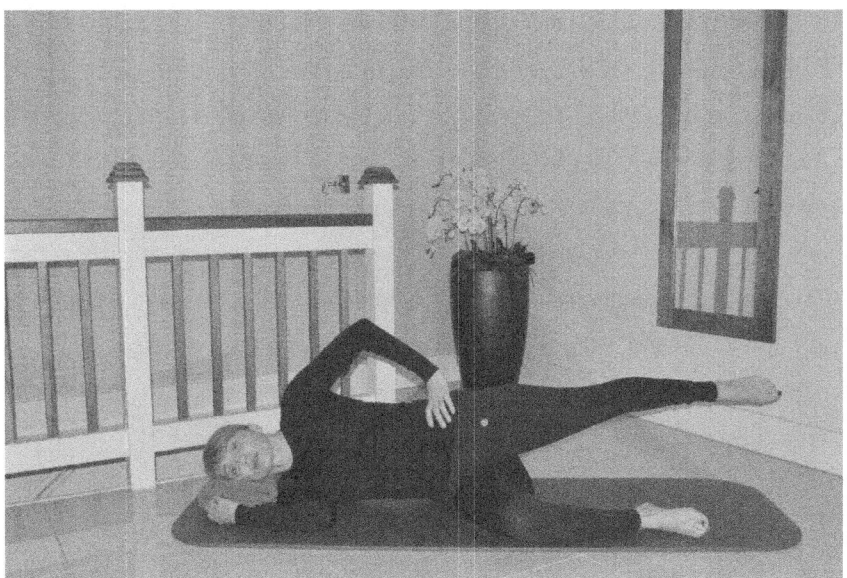

Hypermobility Without Tears

Side lying exercises are important for balance. These exercises allow us to play with balance in a supported way. When we lie on our sides, we have little contact with the ground. This means our proprioception will be challenged too. Once you have assumed your position, spend some time sensing the contact points into the floor. The more familiar you are, the easier the balance element of this exercise is going to be.

Begin with the legs bent as though you were seated on a chair. Then, extend the top leg out until it is straight and in line with the body. It should be as though you were standing on one leg upright.

The aim here is to be able to facilitate a gentle swinging motion of the top leg forward and backwards of the midline without the spine being disturbed. Begin to roll the leg forwards as you inhale – the thigh bone has the ability to roll and sink into the hip socket. The feeling is of the thigh bone articulating in the pelvis, but the challenge is great because the leg is long and we are on our side. As the leg swings forward, we aim not to flex the spine or arch the back.

The leg that is resting on the floor has just as an important role as the leg that is moving. It needs to stay heavy into the floor. Without this element, the mobile leg will not be allowed full freedom. Let go of the underneath leg and spine to free up the top leg.

Chapter Five: Balance

As you exhale, roll the thigh bone backwards, until the hip is extended but the back is not arched. There will be a response from the lumbar spine, but it should not overextend.

Notice the rolling action of the thigh bone forward and backward. Think of the alignment of the leg so that the leg is parallel to the floor and the foot is not dropping down towards the floor. Try to keep the leg at hip height the whole journey forward and back. Keep sending the breath down the leg to continuously create space and freedom in the joints.

Repeat on the other side. Does one side feel different than the other?

EXERCISE – Standing Hip Roll

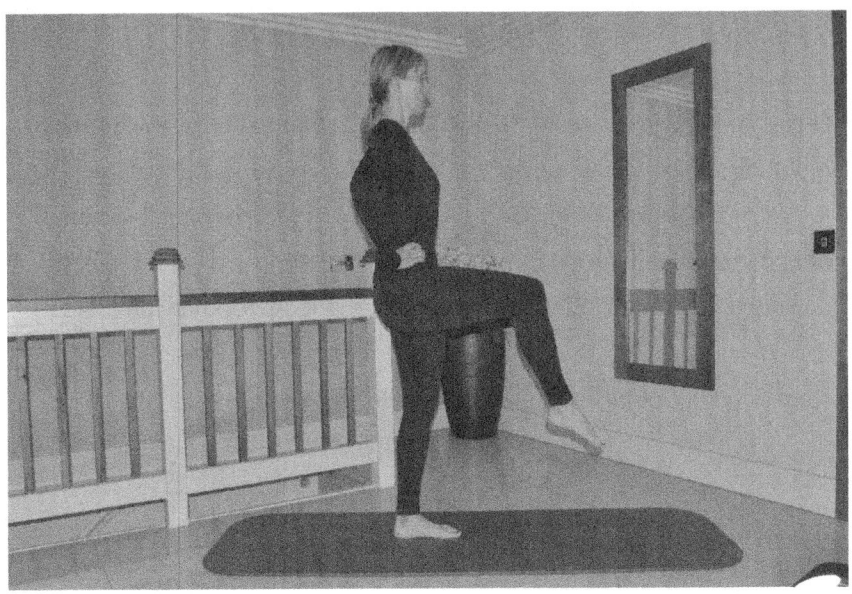

If we have spent time establishing the weightiness of our feet and lower limbs, our ability to stand on one leg will be much improved. As with the exercise above, we must release the static limb into the ground to allow the moving limb freedom. The static leg is your stability here.

You can hold on to a chair if you have any balance disorders.
Assume a standing posture and feel the legs being drawn down into the ground. As you exhale, allow one leg to become heavier. Focus on the weight of that leg. As that leg becomes heavier, can you allow the other leg to become lighter, so much so that it begins to float up from the

Chapter Five: Balance

floor? Allow the head of the thigh bone to rest in the pelvis – feel the weight of the thigh bone and the lightness of the knee. It is like a pendulum – one end swings down giving lightness to the other end. Do you feel the need to arch or round your back? If so, try to establish more weight into your tailbone. It is important to check the standing knee joint does not hyperextend. This is common as we use this as our stability – but it is a false stability. Utilising the knee joint at this stage will make us very vulnerable to injury and fall. Think how this translates to walking or climbing stairs.

Hold the position with an inhale, returning the leg to the floor on the exhale. Aim for a slow, controlled lowering of the leg which then allows the foot to settle back into the floor. As balance is established, we are then in a position to try the other leg with minimum disruption to our posture.

Repeat on the other leg and take time to notice any differences.

Through these exercises, can you start to feel the feet supporting you in everyday life? If you can do so without causing pain, try to walk barefoot at home as much as possible. This trains the muscles and builds sensory awareness.

Once we start to notice and feel the feet in motion, walking is going to start to feel more comfortable. Please remember that it is going to be expected to feel post-exercise muscle soreness, especially if you have not worked the feet before. These muscles need training, like any other muscle.

How can we translate this foundational work into the dynamics of walking? Walking is a whole body movement. I would love everyone to enjoy walking – even if it's only 10 steps to begin with. Let's try a barefoot mindful walking exercise at home or on safe ground.

Try not to force your walk – it needs to be natural with the no strain, no pain approach. Key points to look out for:

- Strike the floor heel first so that you flex your ankle.
- For ideal foot position, try to strike with the outside edge of the heel.
- Allow the rest of the foot to roll as you travel forwards, making the big toe last to hit the ground.
- The big toe is also the last point of contact as you propel forward.
- Importantly allow the arms to gently swing in opposition to the legs thereby creating a rotation in the torso.
- Keep the gaze forward.

It may feel strange or awkward to begin with, especially if you have not been allowing your upper body to join in the walk. We need to promote a counter-rotation between the pelvis and the ribcage – so that all the tissues are being loaded and are gliding with every step. If we adopt a

Chapter Five: Balance

static torso in walking – often the case when we have been in pain – it actually leads to more pain long term. Structures become stuck, tissue becomes sticky rather than fluid. Allow the pelvis to move when you walk – enjoy a gentle wiggle of the hips. I have worked with people who have been told to keep their pelvis still when walking. This is a mystery to me – unless there was too much lateral tilt in the pelvis when walking, which can put strain on the surrounding muscles. The pelvis is designed to tilt, rotate and laterally shift with each step. But with a hypermobile body, we do need to keep the range of control too.

Incorporate gentle walking practice into your movement therapy program until it begins to feel the norm. Notice how you start to move like this in everyday walking.

This whole body movement is a crucial element of building a dynamic movable structure. We are going to look at the concept of biotensegrity and elasticity in our following chapter – Posture.

Chapter Six: Posture
An Awakening of the Senses

"Tensegrity demonstrates the natural balance of forces, the dynamic tension network, and an integrated movement system that is applicable to all living things."
Graham Scarr, Author – Biotensegrity. The Structural Basis of Life, 2018

Posture completes our journey. Posture is not something that can be taught in a mechanical way – rather it will emerge from all the work you have invested in so far through this book. People are often taught to stand up straight, pull the shoulders back, do not slouch. These are all just mechanical instructions to our brain. This does not talk effectively to a dynamic sensory system that makes us who we are. Our sensory awareness has to be involved in our posture. Posture cannot be 'fixed' or 'static' like a soldier on duty. Neutral is just a concept – it does not exist in movement. Posture needs to be dynamic, changeable and elastic. With a dynamic posture, your body becomes responsive to its environment. It changes with you, with the demands you place upon it. It reacts appropriately to the ground force and gravity.

Hypermobility Without Tears

In order to fully sense how this works, we need to touch on the subject of biotensegrity.

The IMM philosophy is to remove a *no pain, no gain* attitude and replace it with a *no pain, no strain* approach. If we attempt to fix our posture mechanically, this is going to cause stress and tension in the body. Importantly, it is not a long-term strategy either. Your body would be so tired with the excess effort required to keep that fixed posture perfect, there is a high chance you would give it up. We have been working through this book to unwind tension, reflect on how our body feels and re-program our movement patterns. When we have lived with chronic pain, or the fear of it, our nervous systems adapt. They turn to 'fight or flight' mode – the anticipation of danger. We mentioned earlier in the book about central sensitization – it is part of this process of living on red alert.

By taking time to really listen to our body, finding the mental stillness to tune into our sensory awareness we start to operate from a restorative place. We reveal a freer, lighter version of our previous self. A body that can feel the connections within the body, a mind that responds without fear and with pleasure of movement.

Robert Schliep, an anatomist and fascia expert, states "there is no need for extraneous, unnecessary tightness, floppiness or strain". That is how we can move dynamically when we tune in, work with our fascia and our whole integrated body.

Chapter Six: Posture

We need our connective tissue to be elastic, where it has the ability to bounce back from movement. With our collagen defects, this is invariably a longer process than with a 'normal' tissue make up, but it is achievable. Small steps are required, paced appropriately and regularly. Little and often is the key to starting. Schliep mentions that we need a suitable balance between stiffness (resistance to deformation) and elasticity (the ability to reform the original shape). Take a spring, for example. You can pull it and it expands. It has tension placed upon it. This is not a bad thing – it is essential for our muscle movement. When you release the spring, it has enough 'good tension' to bounce back to its original length without experiencing damage or injury. This is healthy movement. But a problem occurs if you keep pulling on the spring beyond its natural range. In fact, you strain it so much that the spring loses its natural bounce, the shape changes and it is no longer functional. That's a poor movement strategy. We aim to be light, bouncy and responsive to force.

Imagine your body is filled with many springs, all expanding outwards pressing in multiple directions. There is enough 'good tension' created in the body to create your shape and make it bouncy too. It is this good tension that creates our posture. We need tension in the body – it keeps us upright. Without it, we would collapse like a sack of potatoes. Tensegrity is a self-organizing, load-distributing and low-energy structure. We use less energy and strain to maintain our structure when we start to appreciate the human body in this way.

Hypermobility Without Tears

Biotensegrity explains how the bones on either side of a joint can remain completely stable yet move with the minimum of effort, and how the soft tissues are able to guide them. (Scarr, 2018). Scarr refers to the tensional network as an 'automatic shifting suspension complex'

Let's experience these forces in movement.

EXERCISE – Quadruped Arm and Leg

Assume a quadruped position, as we learnt in our chapter on Stability. If we are now comfortable supporting ourselves, the next step would be to challenge this position. Rather than thinking of this as an exercise of attempting to lift the opposite arm and leg, let's re-examine this exercise in light of the biotensegrity model.

I often explain this concept to my clients through the analogy of an inflatable snowman at Christmas. When you first start to inflate these objects are flat, but as the air enters the snowman starts to expand. It will not expand in a linear fashion because the air would travel everywhere in multiple directions. The snowman would start to take shape as the air pressure pushes out against all available surfaces. Eventually, the snowman would be fully inflated and its shape would be understandable to all. The 'posture' of the snowman was not created with rigidity and fixing. It was created from internal pressure – I refer to

Chapter Six: Posture

it as 'good pressure'. We do need a certain amount of pressure inside the body otherwise we would collapse on the floor like the deflated snowman. It makes sense therefore that if we are trying to 'fix' our posture and 'stand up straight' this is going to inevitably put stress in the body. We are fighting the natural 'good pressure' we have inside. Try to stand for a moment and feel the sensation of the inflatable snowman – the pressure expanding your body in multiple directions. Think of this pressure travelling in all directions – do not try to stand up straight and linear. Think 3-dimensional posture.

From a quadruped position imagine the body expanding. The arm and leg begin to expand along the floor (keep them touching the floor to begin with). Rather than thinking of lifting the limbs off the floor, think of them continuing to expand – they have nowhere to go except up into the air. The limbs almost float up because of this expansion of space inside the body, like we are being inflated.

Your whole body takes part in this exercise – as opposed to individual limbs being lifted by hip and shoulder joints. Feel how you can use your breath to create the inflation of the body – really breathe into the shape and grow. It is less stressful and puts less strain on individual joints. We actually become more powerful working this way.

Hypermobility Without Tears

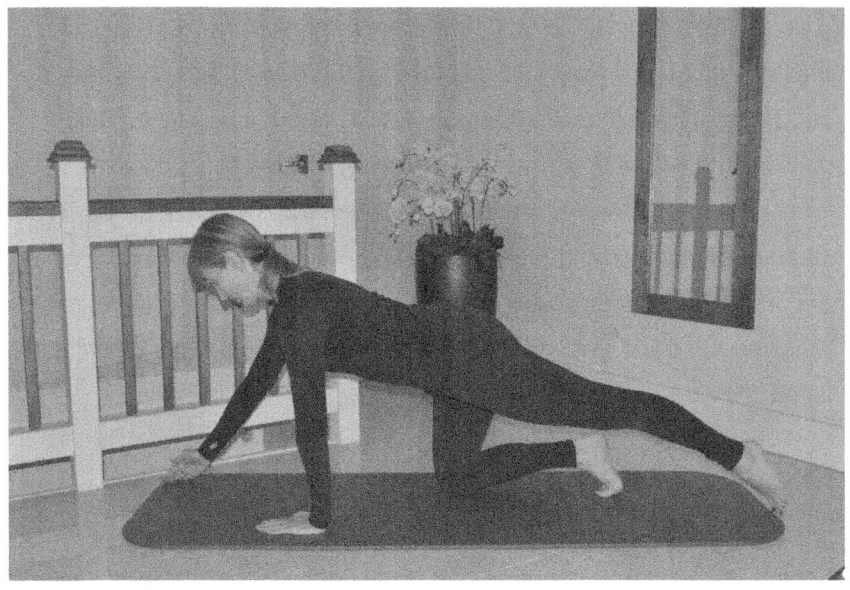

Photo a) demonstrates the expansion of the body in multiple directions.

Chapter Six: Posture

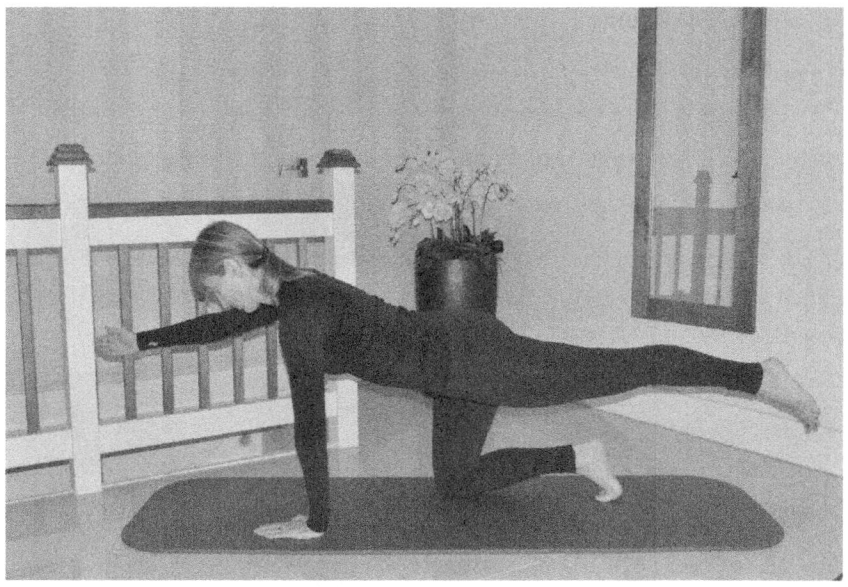

Photo b) demonstrates the body continuing to expand – until the limbs float up.

EXERCISE – Plank

This can be a more challenging exercise – make sure you are happy with all the quadruped variations before moving onto this exercise. I like to use this as an example of the biotensegrity model in action. How can we take a challenging movement and make it fluid? We can if we are tuning into our tensegrity. Assume the idea of the snowman again.

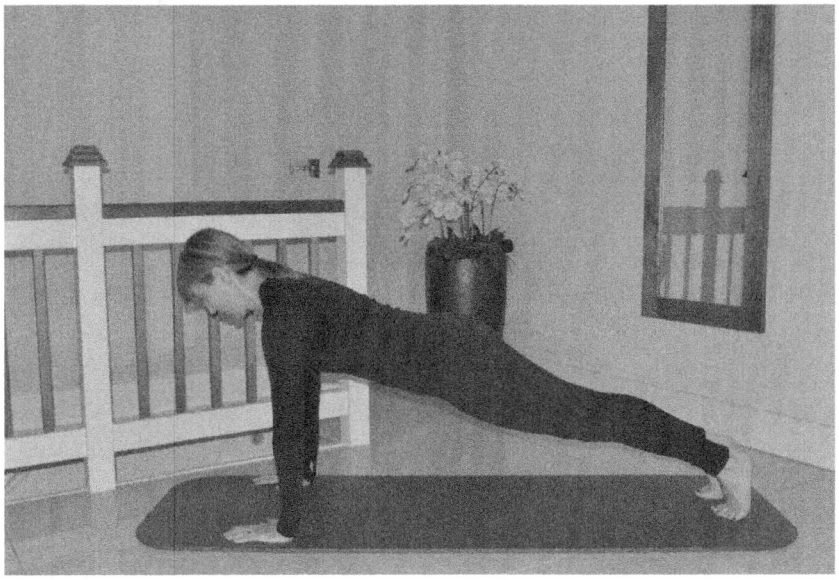

From a quadruped position, slide one leg out behind you. Tuck the toes under for support. Feel the arms reaching down into the ground, the head reaching in the opposite direction to the extended leg. With an exhale, can you expand the other side of your body so that the second leg expands out along the floor to meet the other one? Keep expanding

Chapter Six: Posture

the body down into the ground and up away from the ground simultaneously. Take one breath before returning to the quadruped position and rest.

EXERCISE – Side Plank Variations

Again, I use this example to demonstrate how movements may become challenging and yet with the correct organisation we can access them. I've included three movements with photos here – one seated, one kneeling and one on the feet. We use exactly the same principles as for the plank, except now all the expansion is going down through one side of the body. This is great for building lateral strength and control. Before attempting this exercise, please make sure you are comfortable with the side lying exercise and standing on one leg exercise. We also need a good understanding of our shoulder stability. With less contact with the floor, the proprioceptive requirements are going to be higher than before.

Feel the pressure drop through one hand and one sit bone, knee or foot depending on the version. As you expand down into the ground, can you allow the body to expand upwards at the same time?

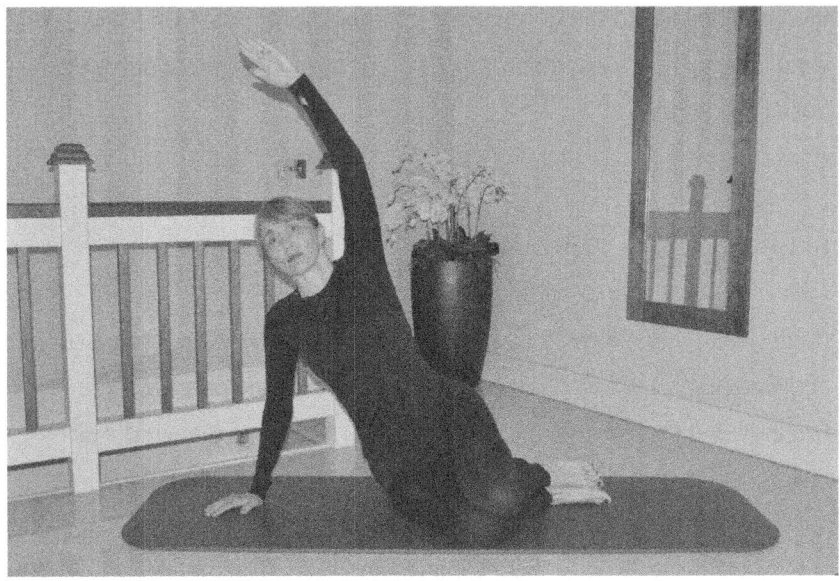

Seated version of side weight-bearing.

Start sitting as shown in the photo, with one hand on the floor to support your weight. This can be challenging to begin with, as we need to be able to support our own body weight with one arm. The shoulder organisation on the supporting arm is important, so that the shoulder does not rise up to the ear. As you support yourself, allow the opposite arm to float up and lean gently to the side. At this stage, do not attempt to lift the pelvis off the ground. Can you have the sense of the weight dropping down into the ground through the arm and the legs? This can free up the opposite arm to float up above the head. Notice the waist stays long on both sides of the body. If you allow the waist to shorten, you will collapse downwards.

Chapter Six: Posture

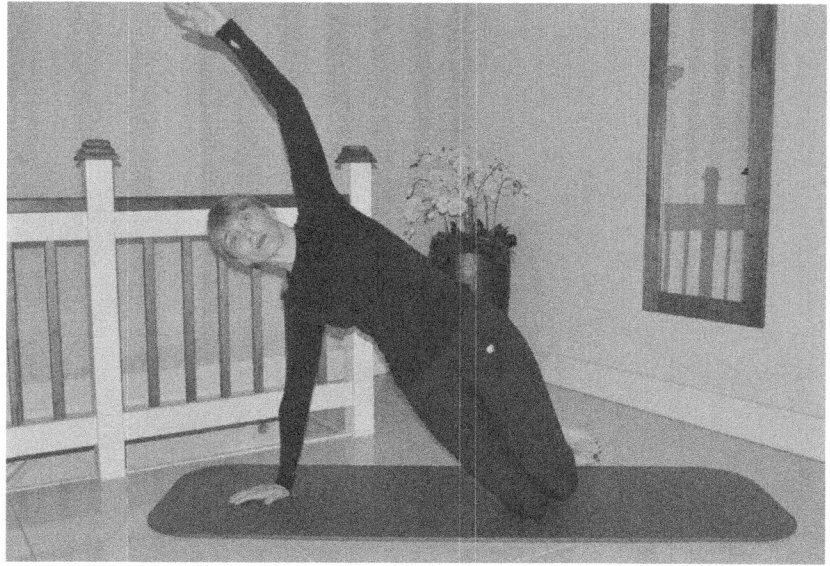

Kneeling version of side weight-bearing.

This version will require greater awareness and strength of the supporting arm, but the same theory applies. Start seated as in the first photo. As the weight drops down through the arm and the legs, can the pelvis become lighter and float up off the floor? Feel a continuous line from the floating arm down to the pelvis. They are connected. Do not worry if your pelvis does not lift as high to begin with. It is most important that we do not strain to lift the body up. Start small and build up strength.

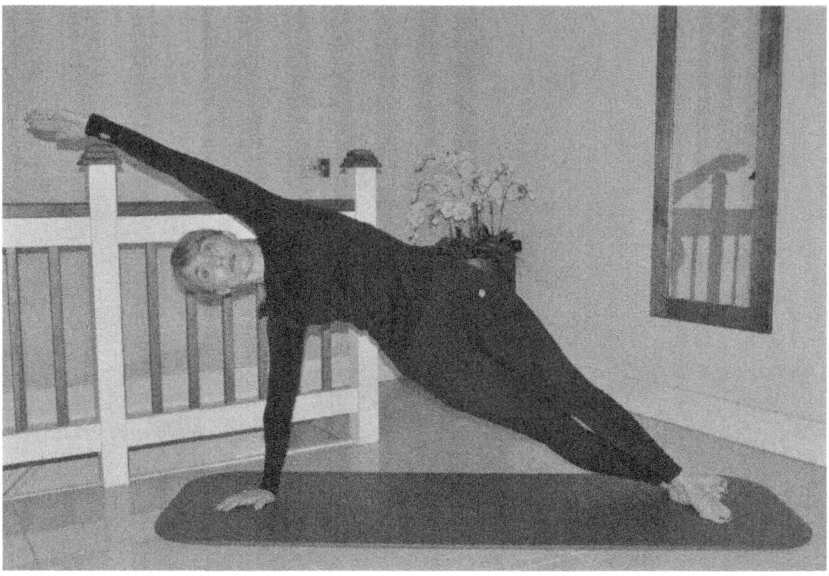

Standing version of side weight-bearing.

This advanced version requires full-body organisation and the felt sense of the 'inflatable snowman' idea in your own body. Please ensure you are comfortable with the kneeling version before you move onto this version.

Once again, start seated but with the top leg in front of the underneath leg. The feet are touching each other. As the knees and pelvis are now going to come off the floor, the feet and hand are going to be supporting the body. Allow the weight to drop down through the arm and the feet to lift the pelvis and torso up. There must be a sense of travelling away

Chapter Six: Posture

from the feet to allow the legs to straighten. Once in position, feel the expanding pressure in multiple directions – down through the hand, down through the feet, out of the crown of the head and out through the free arm. The whole structure is fully supported by the idea of the biotensegrity. Our energy moves down and up simultaneously.

When you finish the movement, slowly lower yourself back down. Going down is as important as going up – we need to work the muscles both ways. Try not to collapse down onto the floor. It is not necessary to hold these positions – this will save strain and tension in the body. Instead move in and out of them smoothly and fluidly.

You can apply the biotensegrity theory to any movement in everyday life.

EXERCISE – Getting Out of a Chair

This is often a troublesome movement for many people. It often causes back discomfort and we feel the need to over use the arms to help us out of a chair. But, if we've been following all the exercises and theories in this book – we now know that it is our contact point through our feet that is going to get us out of any chair. With the biotensegrity model, the feet expand down into the floor and just like the snowman expanding up into the air, we also rise up into the air from the chair. The more pressure we can place into the feet, the easier it is for the pelvis to float up out of the chair. It is okay to hinge forward slightly when you do this. Importantly, if you use your legs, you will be less inclined to use your lower back.

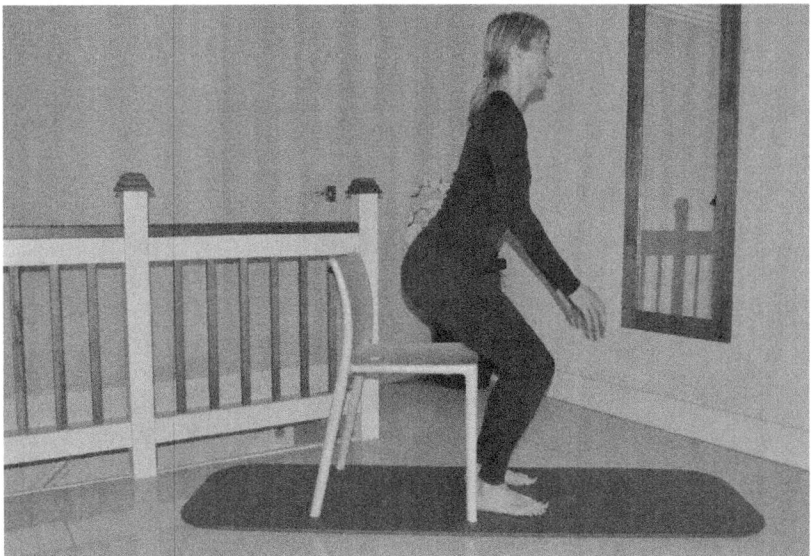

Chapter Six: Posture

EXERCISE – Climbing Stairs

An everyday occurrence for many of us, but yet one which can cause such pain. Let's try to apply the biotensegrity model to this movement too, to make our everyday activities easier.

As you place your first foot on the step, the pressure needs to drop down through the whole surface of the foot. This contact with the ground through the foot should activate the glutes. The glutes and the feet working together have the power to lift your whole body up onto the next step. Sometimes we can allow ourselves to collapse into the front leg causing knee and hip pain. We then have to drag the rest of the body up the step. If we use the ground force to press down and be pushed up at the same time, it will make this movement much easier.

Hypermobility Without Tears

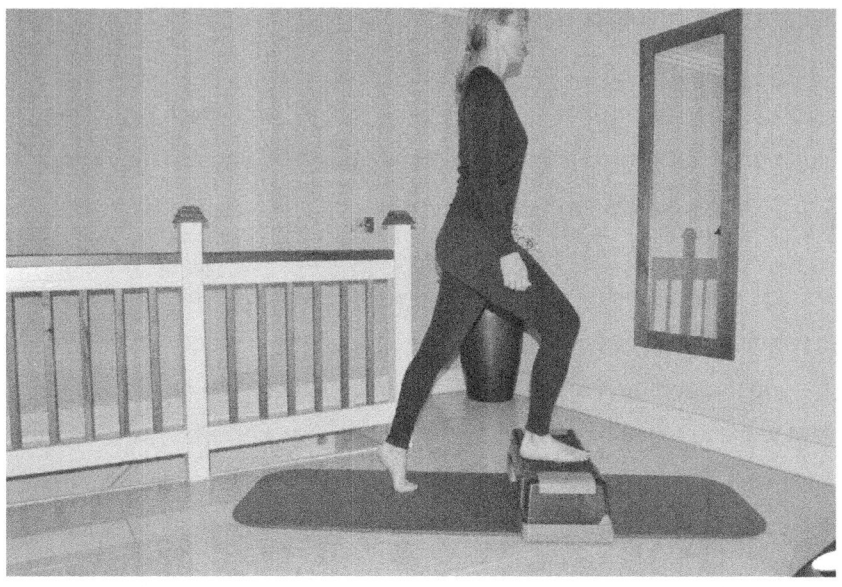

Photo a) – allow the pressure to drop down into the front foot.

Chapter Six: Posture

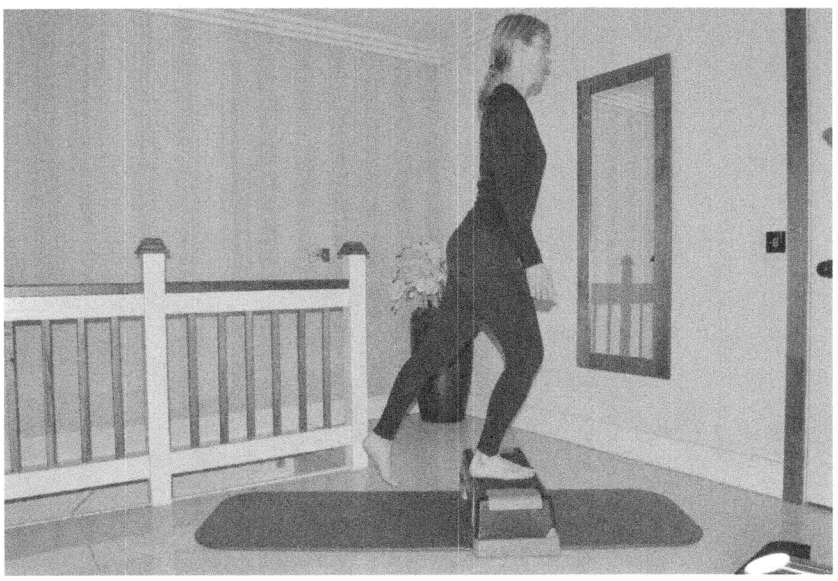

Photo b) – power up through the front leg to lift the body up.

Our standing posture becomes automatically impacted by this theory of how the human body works. Without the stress of trying too hard to find the perfect posture, can we find a quiet place to discover our own tensional network?

Hypermobility Without Tears

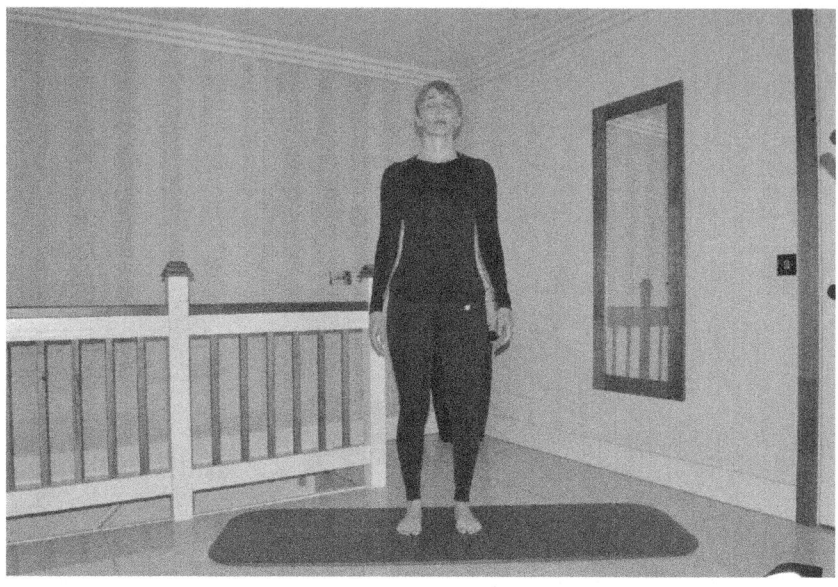

We are seeking softness through the body – joints, skin, surfaces and organs. But with the understanding of the biotensegrity model and ground force, can we allow the body to feel the support from underneath? Our objective is to find a 'quiet place' without tension.

If we can establish this, we are able to make everyday tasks like lifting and carrying easier too. In this standing arm roll exercise with small weights (you could use any object here, but I would not recommend making it too heavy to start with) find your feet first. Allow the weight of the feet and the legs to give freedom to the arms. The weight that I am carrying is fully supported from the pelvis down into the ground. I am in reality not lifting the weight with my shoulders or arms, but with my whole body. The 'I' in the IMM stands for Integral because it is designed

Chapter Six: Posture

to integrate the whole body so it works as one unit, rather than through disjointed parts.

EXERCISE – Standing Arm Roll with Weights

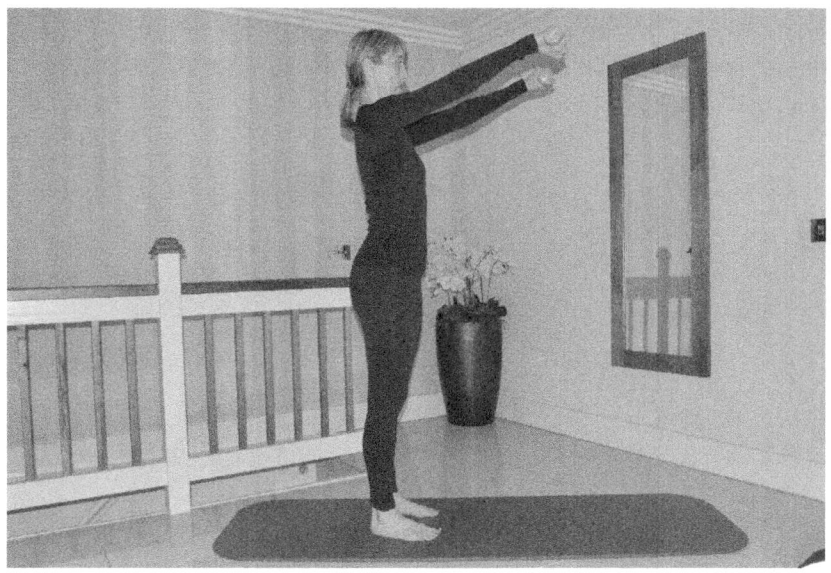

Photo a) demonstrates correct lifting posture.

When we are presented with carrying weights, even our shopping bags or lifting our children, the integrity of the whole system is essential to prevent injury. Notice in the photo above how the ribs stay directly above the pelvis while lifting weights. It is important to connect with the feet heavy into the ground. This will activate the leg muscles, which in turn will support the lifting action. Try to lift the weight from your feet, not from your shoulders.

Photo b) highlights a common error made when lifting a weight. Without integrity of the whole system, the weight forces the ribcage to shift backwards in relation to the pelvis. You can see from the photo that the lumbar spine is a clear area of force and is could result in discomfort and pain.

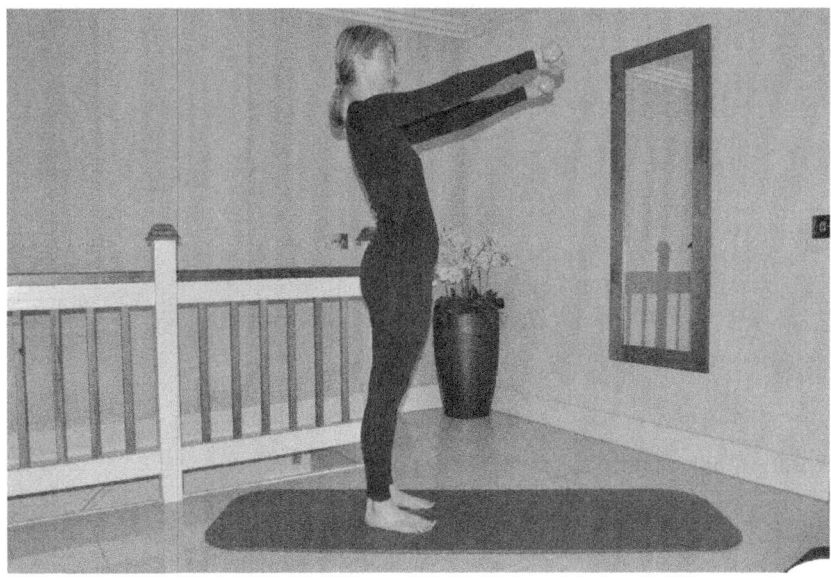

Photo b) demonstrates poor lifting action.

Chapter Six: Posture

Now that we have explored the 6 elements of the movement strategy for a hypermobile body, let's look at some of the positive changes we can look forward to in the following chapter.

Chapter Seven: Practical Improvements with the IMM

"This gives me strength and stability. My body feels amazing and connected after class."
Nicole, hEDS client

I hope you have been following along with the movements in the book and have noticed some changes already. As a longstanding chronic pain sufferer with hypermobile EDS, I can look back and reflect on how this work has really helped me and my clients. I wanted to share with you my top list of benefits that we can expect to enjoy by regular participation.

- *Increased sensory awareness*
  Spending time listening to our body and mind.

- *Strength and control of range of movement*
  Learning how to control range of movement with reduced injury and building strength.

Hypermobility Without Tears

- *Improved muscle tone = less pain*
  The more we move, the more toned our tissue becomes. That means less pain.

- *Decrease in pain and confident self-management techniques*
  As above, but feeling self-confident too that we are doing the right thing.

- *Injury prevention / decrease subluxations*
  All of the above – it starts to impact at multi-level.

- *Improved breathing patterns*
  Taking time to re-learn how to breathe efficiently and effectively for whole body health.

- *Dynamic posture with stamina*
  Understanding of the inner tensional workings of the body will create a resilient posture.

- *'Good tension' in the body, not unhelpful tension*
  Biotensegrity in action.

- *Overall quality of life – energy, vitality, ability*
  With less pain and more confidence in exercising regularly energy levels rise.

Chapter Seven: Practical Improvements with the IMM

- *Confidence, mood and stress levels*
  When energy levels rise, we feel good! Stress decreases.

- *Sense of overall wellbeing and calm*
  Whole body health – feeling good inside and out.

- *Clearer thoughts and less brain fog*
  Exercising helps to clear the mind and aids focus.

- *Sleep hygiene*
  With increased activity and reduced stress, sleep quality improves.

- *Community and support*
  Being part of something has a huge impact on wellbeing. Exercising with others or finding a therapist or teacher who really understands hypermobility is amazing.

This book has covered in detail my six essential principles to build a healthy, resilient hypermobile body. Through practicing my Integral Movement Method (IMM) you will to learn and embody these elements in a methodical way. It is designed to work on your mind and body so that you start to feel connected and in control. The method is particularly useful in terms of building proprioception, sensory awareness, training appropriate breathing patterns and the ability to recognise when you are holding muscular tension.

The IMM is based on my own research into mind-body connections, into the science of the mind and movement. It is the foundation of all my work with my clients and has helped many people with their hypermobility and chronic pain. It has a scientific base and is accessible and easy to follow. My method will teach you to recognise signs of stress and tension in your body, it will change your physiology and will begin to build important mind- body connections that are often weaker in a hypermobile body due to reduced proprioception.

Let's examine why the method works so well for hypermobility and EDS.

There are 5 steps to my Integral Movement Method:

- Unwind

- Explore

- Assess

- Refine

- Reflect

Chapter Seven: Practical Improvements with the IMM

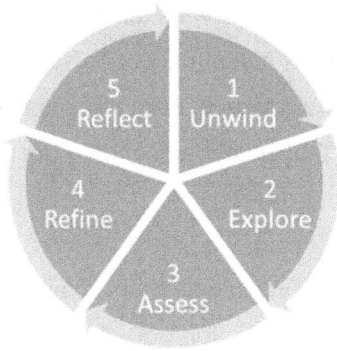

1. Unwind

Hypermobility often causes muscular pain. As we have been discussing earlier in the book, hypermobility can allow the individual to stretch more or do more without realising that soft tissue strain is taking place, due to the lack of body awareness. It is not until later, when the pain arrives, that we realise what we have done. There is also the issue of muscular tension caused by poor postural habits or repetitive actions in our daily life. If there is anxiety and stress related to the condition, this can cause tension, which leads to muscle pain. It becomes a vicious circle. The more we worry about our pain, the more the muscles tense and the more pain signals are sent out by the brain. We need to disrupt that pattern before we can even get to the pain. The Unwind section of the IMM is vital to this. This is where we start to unwind and let go of muscular and mental nervous tension that may have built up in the body that day (or longer if you have been suffering from stress and pain for some time). It also starts to build the essential proprioception, or body awareness, so that we become more conscious of our actions and movements.

These are a few moments when we close our eyes, observe our breath and switch off our thinking brain. It is your time to stop and be aware of your body. We lead busy lives, our brains are stimulated from the moment we wake up. It is time to notice your body and whether you are aware of what I refer to as 'holding patterns'. Are you breathing softly and rhythmically? Even our breath can be disrupted by our pain thoughts. Maybe you are holding your breath? Are you able to totally surrender to the floor and allow your body to melt into the ground?

Through the process of unwinding, you immediately start to release the tension from the mind and body that you may not have been aware of during the day. You allow your bones, tissues and organs to soften and start creating the space your body and mind crave. It's time to stop fighting and allowing your body to let go a little. The more you can notice your body and its own weight resting on the floor, the greater your degree of proprioception.

Chapter Seven: Practical Improvements with the IMM

2. Explore

Explore means it is time to start moving. Movement will not be hurried or forced. It may be as slow and gentle as you require, but I encourage you to begin to move – as long as you listen to your body. This program is where we explore soft, slow and mindful movements – exploring and exposing resistance and tension you may be holding onto. You are exploring your body's potential, your feelings, your power of focus and concentration. It is time for movement meditation. It is most important that, as a hypermobile client, our new mantra becomes 'it's not about the range, it's about the control'. It is preferable to do smaller, controlled movements well within the potential full range as opposed to move to end of range. If we move to end of range, we will not learn joint stability. For a hypermobile client, this can be the hardest concept of all – reigning it back in! Once we learn control, we can start to build back in ranges of movement.

3. Assess

We will be assessing throughout the program – when we pause to re-evaluate. This stage is therefore a chance to assess whether you are in fact moving without strain, or you have reverted to an old movement pattern. Have you been thinking about control, or have you been pushing to your biggest range? We pause, we wait, we observe, we shift our mental focus from outside to inside the body. If we are moving in a forceful or distracted way, we are creating more tension in the body.

A typical example would be to clench the jaw muscles in tension, or shoulders rising up to the ears causing neck and shoulder discomfort. Or maybe we have stopped breathing altogether.

So a pause, a reassessment is a chance to check in with yourself. If you have been clenching your jaw, it's okay. You just need to recognise that, bring attention to it.

4. Refine

After the pause, we get moving again. We have learnt something neurologically in that assessment – maybe now your jaw muscles will stay soft, your shoulders will drape down your back, and your breath will be quiet, deep and full. We continue with the exercises exploring all ranges of movement suitable for us, but continuing to observe the body as a whole. We want to observe our body in an integrated way.

5. Reflect

Reflect is an important phase of the program – we require that your brain notices if your body feels different. Compare how you felt at the

Chapter Seven: Practical Improvements with the IMM

beginning of the class to how you feel now. You may feel calmer, quieter, and sleepy. You may feel energised and free. You may feel connected and stronger in your centre. What is most important is that you have taken the time to register that something has shifted – mentally and physically. If we skip this stage, we miss a vital opportunity to connect and accept change in awareness into the body. We are retraining the brain and our nervous system to accept this change, to allow you to build confidence that it is safe and okay to move. Controlled movement does not harm or cause damage, but it is vital to your overall health and wellbeing.

****

I do hope you have found this book to be a useful companion in your journey to moving well, moving more and enjoying movement. Remember, it is all about the small steps. Every small physical step you take will have a massive emotional impact. This is vital to our recovery and our road to health. I truly wish you well along this often unpredictable road. You are not alone in your journey. Keep strong.

I wish to thank you for taking time to read my journey and I hope it has given you hope that no matter what EDS or hypermobility decides to throw at you, there is hope. These conditions by nature are unpredictable, frustrating and isolating. One of my desires for myself and for you is to never let these conditions define us or stop us achieving what we want to do. The journey to health and wellbeing can be bumpy sometimes, but these ups and downs give us the opportunity to develop resilience and inner strength. Harness that.

As Glinda the Good Witch says in the film The Wizard of Oz:

"You always had the power, my dear. You just had to learn it for yourself"

Yours in movement.

Jeannie

Further Information

Jeannie Di Bon is available for one-to-one sessions and Skype sessions. She can also be contacted should your group or organisation wish her to speak at an event or run a training session on movement therapy. Remember to follow her on social media for regular tips and exercise ideas for the EDS and hypermobile community.

Email jeannie@jeanniedibon.com or visit www.jeanniedibon.com

If you like what you've read, join the online platform for safe, effective exercise programmes designed specifically for those with hypermobility, EDS and chronic pain.

THE 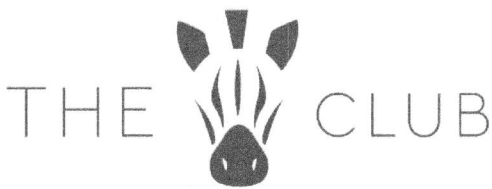 CLUB

Visit www.jeanniedibon.com/products to find out more.

References

Butler et al, 2003, Explain Pain, Noigroup Publications.

Byrnes et al, 2017, Is Pilates an effective rehabilitation tool? A systematic review, Elsevier.

Clayton et al, 2015, Proprioceptive precision is impaired in Ehlers-Danlos Syndrome, Springerplus

Cruz-Diaz et al, 2017, The effectiveness of 12 weeks of Pilates intervention on disability and kinesiophobia in patients with chronic low back pain, Sage Journals.

Golman et al, 1993, Mind Body Medicine – How to use your mind for better health, New York Consumers Report Book.

Lederman, E, 2008, The myth of core stability, Elsevier Science Direct.

McNeil et al, 2017, The Pilates client on the hypermobility spectrum, Elsevier

Morgan et al, 2007, Asthma and airways collapse in two heritable disorders of connective tissue, Annals of the rheumatic diseases.

Parry, J, 2017, Dislocation / Subluxation Management, https://www.ehlers-danlos.com/dislocation-subluxation-management/, The EDS Society Global Learning Conference, Las Vegas.

Scaravelli, V, 1991, Awakening the Spine, Pinter & Martin.

Scarr, G, 2018, Biotensegrity. The Structural Basis of Life, Handspring Publishing Ltd.

Schliep, R, 2015, Fascia in Sport and Movement, Handspring Publishing.

Todd, M, 1937, The Thinking Body, New York Dance Horizons.

Van Der Kolk, B, 2014, The Body Keeps the Score.

www.mastcellaction.org – Mast Cell Activation Disorder.

Made in the USA
Las Vegas, NV
25 March 2024

87756245R00085